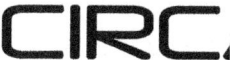

Nutritional Guide to CIF

CW01558771

CIRC

DIET

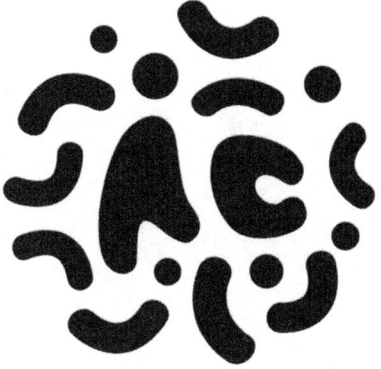

DR. AYSEGUL CORUHLU

CIRCADIAN DIET by Dr. Aysegul Coruhlu, MD. PhD

About the Author

Dr. Aysegul Coruhlu was born July 4, 1969. She completed her secondary education in Izmir and graduated from the Istanbul Faculty of Medicine in 1994. While specializing in biochemistry at Sisli Etfal Hospital, she studied for her master's program in biomedical engineering at Bosphorus University.

Dr. Coruhlu began to work as a biochemist at the American Hospital in 2000. She later became the head of the Intermed Polyclinic Laboratory. Dr. Coruhlu also received training at the American Anti-Aging Academy.

She was one of the first to implement advanced anti-aging approaches such as antioxidant tests, tests measuring the speed of aging, hormone and genetic tests, the alkaline diet, prescribing tailor-made vitamin and mineral boosts, and intravenous antioxidant applications.

Dr. Coruhlu has focused on preserving health at the cell level.

The author has published two more books, *Alkali Diyet* ("The Alkaline Diet") and *Tokuz ama Açız* ("We are Full yet Hungry").

Contents

About the Author 3

Introduction 7

How to Use This Book? 17

Our Circadian Clock 22

The Ultimate 5 51

Chapter 1: 53

Chapter 2: 81

The Food-Disease Connection 90

The Cost of an Unhealthy Diet 98

Chapter 3: 113

Chapter 4: 120

Chapter 5: 147

Some Tips So That You Won't Be Bound to Pills All Your Life 176

Epilogue 180

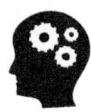

Introduction

"It is not known, for whom time would be a friend, and for whom an enemy."

Time and Humans

Chronos is the god of time in mythology. Time is our most valuable asset, and we can never bring it back. Among all the living creatures, only humans are aware that time on Earth is "limited." Only we humans are aware of our own mortality. On the one hand, this is a type of awareness that causes a tragic confrontation with our own impotence; on the other hand, it sparks a desire to hold on to life to use that time correctly. Humanity has an issue with time. For thousands of years, inventing the time machine, going back in time, ceasing time, and the like, have always been dreams of humans.

We cannot possess time; it slips through our fingers and passes by. For millennia, people assumed that time moved forward in a linear fashion, at a constant pace. But, Einstein proved us wrong. Einstein's "relativity of time" theory won him a Nobel Prize in physics in 1921. Accordingly, time can flow fast or slow, depending on the circumstances. However, in order to really comprehend this difficult theory, we need to have knowledge of complicated technical concepts. Yet, although we cannot completely grasp the relativity of time, we know that it is accurate.

Time, Chronological Time, and "Relativity"

The mentioning of both the Nobel and "time" together in the first paragraph actually summarizes this book, which was inspired by the 2015, 2016, and 2017 Nobel Prizes. The most prestigious award of the scientific world, the Nobel has always been an indicator where science is headed towards. These awards also indicate the future of medicine. Thus, the relevant three studies that were awarded show the most current areas in which medicine is evolving towards. It appears that we should add a new parameter to medicine: the health of our internal biological clocks. Once you finish this book, written as a result of being inspired by these researches, you will see that biological time is also relative.

- You will learn that we have an inner clock.
- You will understand that the incompatibility between our inner clock and our wristwatch can determine our pace of aging.

Are you ready to hear a bold statement?

You will learn to generate your own time machine and discover the secret to aging at your own pace!

Wishing you to always remain "relatively" young…

2017 Nobel Prize in Medicine and Our Biological Clock

In 2017, the Nobel Prize in Medicine was awarded to the discovery of molecular mechanisms controlling the circadian rhythm, namely the biological clock. In the same year, three scientists—Jeffrey C. Hall, Michael Rosbash, and Michael W. Young—received the prize. This is a fairly recent Nobel Prize.

What actually measures the time is not the watch on your wrist; it is the earth. The clock equals the earth. All living beings on Earth adapt to its cycle. Cycles of night and day, of seasons, of climates determine the rules. For millions of years, humans have adapted to these cycles as did all the other species that have survived. Therefore, living in harmony with Earth's clock is a matter of survival. Those who have attuned to the seasons, climates, days, nights have survived and the rest have vanished. The system that provides this harmony is called the "internal biological clock of living beings," or circadian rhythm.

Although we had already known this biological clock existed, the illumination regarding how it actually works occurred with this Nobel Prize. Moreover, this prize also allowed the dawn of a new subfield in medicine—**chronomedicine**—and a new expertise—**chronobiology**. Now, with this book you will take your first step into this realm. You will learn how to wind your internal biological clock.

So…

- What makes the biological clock work?
- What blocks it?
- What happens if the biological clock doesn't work right?
- How can you harmonize the wristwatch on your arm with your biological clock?

Let's begin with the findings of the Nobel-awarded study. The discovery of these three scientists, which is concerned with how the inner clock works, shows us how people synchronize their circadian rhythm to the earth's rhythm. In their study, they first isolated the gene that sustains the daily biological rhythm. They proved that the proteins controlling these genes work in different ways during the day and at night. They found that these biological clock genes are *on* (active) at night and *off* (silent) during the day. The working routine of this internal time was defined as such: "the clock that sets itself every day".

More importantly, this internal time is not all about turning *on* and turning *off*. It also regulates the physiological mechanisms throughout the day. In light of these studies, we now know that the internal clock, namely the circadian rhythm, controls many of the critical functions. For example, our behaviors, hormone levels, sleep patterns, body temperatures, and metabolism as a whole are actually affected by this biological clock.

The overall health of the body is disrupted when the internal time and the external time don't match. In order to help you quickly grasp this mismatch, the best example to illustrate it would be jet lag. Jet lag is the disruption of the inner time in the course of continental flights when we travel to another time zone of the world. If you have experienced jet lag even only once in your life, you would have an idea about how it disrupts your life or your health. Since it's not a frequent experience, it does not create an agenda for health. However, is flying the only reason for the mismatch between internal and external time?

- What about social jet lag?
- What about electronic jet lag?
- What about nutritional jet lag?

What do we have to say about the lifestyle habits that are not in harmony with the body's biological circadian internal clock? We are under the influence of this disharmony every day. Despite the fact that there are hundreds of studies proving the disharmony between the rhythm of life and the biological rhythm as being the cause of many illnesses, accelerated aging, and weight gain, are we going to continue to avoid this matter completely?

It's been only a year and a half since this idea received the Nobel Prize. Therefore, the data and studies are all brand new. That's why I would like for you to read what I have written in this book, underlining sentences as you go along. Why? Because, we either get our acts together right away and set our biological times correctly, or we wait for another five to ten years until the findings of this study are demonstrated not only in textbooks but also on our "streets." You make your decision. It's your time. But, since you bought this book, I assume you have a different perspective. You are at the right place, and you made a great choice. For I will tell you how to spend the following ten years of external time as only five years according to your internal clock. In a manner of speaking, we will develop our own time machines, and we will be the ones to determine the rhythms of our own time. We will get older, but we will not age.

Our Circadian Inner Clock

Observation and curiosity are fundamentals of science. In the eighteenth century, astronomer Jacques d'Ortous observed mimosas. He discovered that the flowers opened their petals toward the sun during the day and closed them at night. Why did mimosas close their petals during the night? Other scientists found out then that animals also reacted differently to light and darkness. They called this alignment with day and night "circadian rhythm." The root of the word circadian is Latin. In Latin *circa* means "about" and *diem* means "day." This is like the *diem* in *carpe diem,* which means "live the day," or "seize the day."

Although how plants, animals, and all living beings adapt to the sun and to the rhythm of the earth has been observed for centuries, the concept of the internal biological clock did not appear until the twenty-first century. Initially, the internal clock genes were discovered in the 1970s. These genes were called *cycle* or *clock* genes. As the names suggest, *ticktock ticktock…*

2015 Nobel Prize: Circadian Rhythm and DNA Repair

The other Nobel Prize regarding time and rhythm is the pride and joy of my country. The study of forty-seven years by the esteemed Turkish-American scientist Aziz Sancar received the Nobel Prize. In actuality, the study consists of many more Nobel-worthy topics. But today, what interests us is his findings regarding circadian rhythm.

Aziz Sancar was doing research on an enzyme called "photolyase." One day, on his way to Turkey for vacation, he sees an article about *jet lag* in Turkish Airlines magazine, which gives him an idea about the relationship between *jet lag* and the circadian rhythm.

The photlyase enzyme that Sancar had been working on for so many years is an enzyme that is activated by light. During his observations, he discovered that visually impaired people and blind mice also have biological functions matching the circadian clock. Sancar had come to the conclusion that we become aware of light through another receptor aside from our eyes. Once he added this data to his prior research, he discovered the proteins CYT 1 and CYT 2. Apparently, our bodies react to sunlight by means of these proteins just like plants react to different wavelengths of light. Therefore, the two proteins are responsible for these reactions.

A year after that flight in 1997, Sancar discovered that these two proteins maintaining the circadian clock were densely situated in two parts of the body. One of them is the retina in the eye, and the other is a part of the brain called suprachiasmatic nucleus—SCN. Even though his publication was impressive, the discovery did not attract enough attention. Nevertheless, Sancar continued with his work.

Until his Nobel-awarded research, Sancar had worked on the circadian clock genes and the correlation between these proteins and DNA repair. He found out that DNA repair is also circadian; in other words, DNA repair occurs at a variety of levels throughout the 24-hour period. Combining this data with the cancer treatment chemotherapy, he came to the following conclusion: "If chemotherapy treatment for cancer takes place at times when DNA repair is insubstantial, chemotherapy would be more effective and more cancer cells can be killed." With this, he won the Nobel Prize.

As a result, between the years 2015 and 2017, research on circadian rhythm became conclusive. Thus, the calibration of the day-night cycle with internal time became evident. As for the word "calibration," it is exactly the right word to be used here. That is to say, there is calibration of the body mechanism to the earth's cycle. We might even call it tuning, perhaps; tuning the cellular rhythm to the earth's rhythm. The aim of this book is exactly that: tuning the rhythm of our cells. If we play out of tune with our environment, then all it will do is to create some cacophony. Harmony is of the essence for music, too.

I have already mentioned that the discovery of the circadian rhythm promoted the development of new sciences such as chronobiology and the birth of a new branch of medicine called chronomedicine. This area of medicine combines all knowledge of the entire medicine world with circadian biology. We connect circadian rhythm with everything we know with regards to living long and healthy and being fit. For all of the functions that you can imagine—eating/being hungry, sleeping/being awake, the rise/decline in hormones, learning/memorizing, repair procedures, detoxification, digestion, maintaining body temperature, growth, aging, reproduction, menopause, all of these functions—are regulated by the circadian clock.

We cannot blame Edison for inventing the light

bulb for the disruption of our system, which has worked according to the cycle of the sun for millions of years, right? All in all, it shouldn't be too difficult to grasp the fact that such behaviors as staying awake until late at night, or eating at odd times are out of tune with our biological internal clock. Edison cannot be the one to blame for that! If you want to put the blame on him and get away with it, do not read this book any further. Give it to someone who would make good use of it.

But if you are willing to create your own time machine at a reasonable book price with no more requirements than a quick and easy-to-understand biochemistry lecture, then you are at the right place. Keep reading. As operatives chasing after new information, let's first set our clocks.

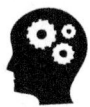

How to Use This Book?

How is it possible that this topic called nutrition still has loose ends? Healthy eating is such a popular topic that almost every month a new book is published, and it always remains on the agenda, globally. There are countless studies proving that the cause of diseases can be traced back to malnutrition, and every day there's a new study that makes such claims. Every day, there is a new publication explaining the correlation between disease and nutrition. There are films, documentaries, and conferences focusing on healthy eating.

I am a member of several clinical institutions abroad. For me, it's essential to obtain the latest data on every area of preventive medicine at conferences organized by these institutions. That's why I frequently participate in these conventions.

However, what I see is that despite the latest technological progress and countless innovations and tens of intriguing scientific publications, nutrition is still at the top of research lists all around the world. It seems that we still haven't reached the required response.

But I Have a Different Approach!

In my opinion, the reason why all this information appears to be variant or inconsistent has a lot to do with the perspective from which we're looking.

- If you approach nutrition through **weight** and **obesity**, you gather the data of a different platform.
- If you approach nutrition with the intention to reduce the risk of diseases related to the internal organs—such as the **heart, liver, brain, intestines—** publications and presentations of this platform grab your attention.
- But if you approach it on a **cellular** basis, or even perhaps on a subcellular-subatomic basis, like myself, you come across an entirely different nutritional approach.

In other words, we get the answer to whatever it is we are looking for. Just like life itself! My objective is to classify and correlate these medical approaches that are mostly accurate and coherent within themselves.

Actually, we doctors find the answers, but you are

at the very beginning of this path. We keep telling you to eat healthy. "You are what you eat" is a phrase instilled in your brain. Every passing day, more and more people depend on advice of experts, read books, and consult the Internet in order to figure out what to do to eat healthy.

Nevertheless, in my opinion, people are still confused about what, when, how, how much, why, and when to eat.

That is exactly what this book is about: it is to quell the confusion in light of all these questions, to install all the data you gathered from different sources into a comprehensible algorithm. This is the fourth book I've written on nutrition. With this book, my goal is to classify the existing data and add to it the missing subject of circadian rhythm.

Now let's have a look at the topics to which you'll find answers in this book:

- Do you know that the time you eat is actually more important than how much you eat?
- Do you know when you should eat?
- Do you know when you shouldn't eat?
- Do you know anything about your biological rhythm?
- What is intermittent fasting?
- Do you truly know why you eat?
- Do you know whether the morsel in your

mouth gives you energy or not?

- How will you know how much you need to eat?
- Do you gain weight only when you overeat?
- Are you aware of the connection between your sleep and your weight?
- How are diseases and nutrition related?
- How is longevity and nutrition related?
- Are your cellular cycles coordinated?
- Does time flow fast or slow for you?
- You may have an unlimited data plan for Wi-Fi; but how about the data plan for life?

As we unveil the answers to all these questions, you will comprehend the connection with our biological clocks. In other words, throughout this book, I will tell you all about the **circadian diet**.

For you to be able to distinguish accurate data from insufficient data regarding nutrition—which is surrounded with excessive input—and get a grasp of the subject as effortless as a doctor, I will examine nutritional biochemistry in the *Ultimate 5* part of this book. I will de-clutter all that mess of knowledge, resembling tangled cables in your head, by replying to the following questions:

Why do we eat?

How much should we eat?

When should we eat?

How should we eat?

What should we eat?

So, I begin with asking the most significant question of this book: **What time does your circadian clock show?**

Our Circadian Clock

"Life is like flowing water, it keeps renewing itself; the body seems to be still, but it constantly changes." —
Rumi

Our biorhythm functions in cycles. It's not fixed. It begins-ends-begins-ends, again and again. Other living beings on Earth also have daily cycles, annual cycles, and biological internal clocks in tune with these cycles. I acknowledge the phrases "cycle" and "flow" as the essence of life. Time is a flowing state: morning-noon-evening, night-day, summer-winter, and years are all cycles.

The sun is the base, the generator of all cycles. The sun sets the earth's clock. The day means that there is sunlight. The night means there is no sunlight. It doesn't matter if the weather is cloudy or even if we do not leave the house, our internal biological clocks distinguish day from night through wavelengths of light. There are biological time receptors in all the cells of our bodies, and they perceive the difference between day and night by wavelengths of light.

If we go into a more detailed description, we can define the setting of our biological clocks according to sunlight as circadian rhythm. Circadian literally means *fluctuation throughout the day*. Throughout the day, all biological activity flows following recurring cycles.

Everything is circadian.

- Hormone secretion is circadian.
- Enzymes become active or passive according to circadian rhythm.
- Metabolic processes occur at different paces throughout the day.
- Body temperature is circadian.
- Digestion is circadian.
- Burning calories/fat is circadian.
- Detoxification of old cells is circadian.
- Whether the DNA repair is good or poor is circadian.
- Actually, every function of every cell is circadian.
- Production and repair procedures take

place at different times. The two cannot be performed simultaneously.

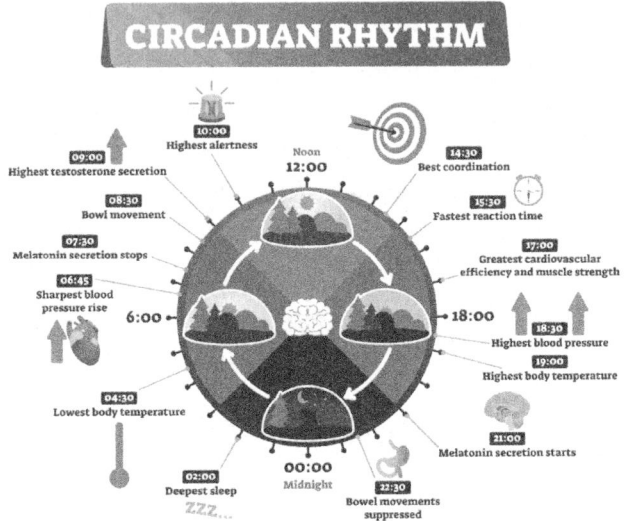

Eating, drinking, your emotional state, hormones, how much you urinate, even your physical stamina are tuned in to these rhythms. Record-breaking Olympic achievements concurring with this rhythm cannot be a coincidence. There are far more Olympic records during early noon hours when the circadian rhythm of humans is at its peak.

The aim of this book is to explain that eating should be circadian. So, let's have a look at the very first question that needs to be answered when talking about eating healthy.

"When do we eat?"

is a far more essential question than
"How much do we eat?"

And the answer is:

We eat according to the circadian rhythm!

Introduction to Circadian Diet

The time for eating is no longer the simple, morning-noon-evening cycle.

The time for eating is about the biological time; in other words, the circadian rhythm. Once you understand the magnitude of the connection between nutrition and the circadian rhythm, you will see that losing weight, eating healthy, remaining fit, and living a long life are not that difficult. **The solution** is as simple as checking what time you eat.

When we talk about nutrition, immediately our troublesome friend the insulin hormone comes to mind. As with all other organs, the functioning of the pancreas, which produces the insulin hormone that adjusts our blood sugar, is circadian. This means that it works more at certain times of the day and less at others. For example, early in the day, the circadian receptors of the pancreas know it's morning and do a better job at adjusting the blood sugar levels. Therefore, the adjustment of the sugar-insulin balance by the pancreas is optimal in the morning.

However, as the day progresses, the biological clock of the pancreas changes. Towards the evening, its ability to balance blood sugar levels decreases. Parallel to the functioning of the pancreas, insulin—similar to all other hormones—is secreted following the circadian rhythm. Just by observing the functioning of the pancreas and the secretion of insulin, we come to the following obvious conclusion: *the pancreas has a strong ability to convert blood sugar into energy in the morning; whereas this ability decreases down to medium ranges around noon and down to low levels in the evening.*

Under the effect of circadian receptors that notice the difference between day and night, the system works towards storing fat in the evening instead of introducing blood sugar into cells and converting it to energy. Because of their increasing tendency towards storing fat, evening meals tend to be transformed into weight, especially causing fat accumulation of the internal organs, even if you eat very little.

In our daily lives, we observe that we gain weight when we eat in the evenings. The science behind this condition is circadian rhythm medicine. We have different circadian metabolisms at night and during the day.

There are several laboratory studies on circadian medicine. For example, one concerns rats left under the sunlight and not allowed to experience the night, who lose their circadian rhythm and as a result quickly gain weight. Another study deals with rats being injected glucose to their bloodstream all day long at the same rate. It was found that balancing their blood sugar was more difficult in the evenings, and consequentially, they would develop type 2 diabetes.

In short, insulin is much better at introducing glucose into the cell to convert it into energy during the day, while it mostly converts it into fat at night.

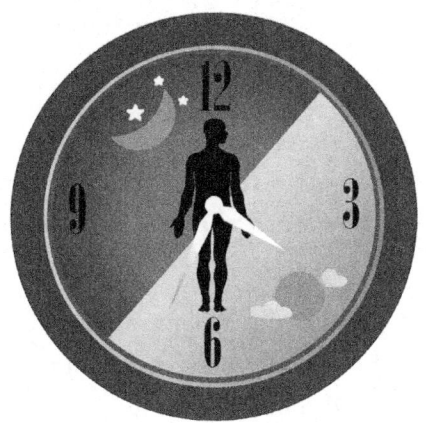

Basically, if we look at the big picture, we see that two separate metabolic processes generate according to the daily cycle.

Catabolic time: daytime functions such as producing energy, mobilization, and burning of calories/fat take place.

Anabolic time: nighttime functions such as preserving energy, storing, growing, and repair take place.

Anabolism and catabolism occur in cycles. Once again, these cycles are grounded in the *survival* mechanism, and their purpose is to use energy in moderation. At night when it is dark and difficult to find food, it is necessary to switch to anabolism for growth, maintenance, repair, and storage in order to prepare for the following day. This is what plants do. During the day, they collect energy from sunlight by photosynthesis and store it in their fruits and roots at night.

Until now, we assumed that the daily insulin quantities were determined solely by blood sugar; now, we know that circadian rhythm also plays an important role in both the quantity and efficiency of insulin.

Not only insulin, but also other hormones are under the influence of the circadian rhythm. Let's put them all aside and focus on the two main hormones that attune our biological internal time to the external time and look at their effects on weight.

The Night Starts with Melatonin. The Morning Alarm Clock Is Cortisol.

Melatonin is the hormone that gives a start to the night segment of the circadian rhythm; while cortisol is the hormone that wakes us up and starts the day segment. These two hormones affect the behavior of insulin and sugar.

Melatonin secretion sends a message to the pancreas that it is nighttime, it is resting time, there is no need for energy, and hence no need for insulin. How does it do that? In the pancreas, there are melatonin receptors.

Towards the morning, as the sun rises, melatonin levels decrease and the opposite hormone of melatonin, cortisol, increases. The cortisol hormone is the "fight or flight" hormone. So, we wake up with a slight increase of the stress hormone. Again, our one-million-year-old survival mechanism wants to prepare us for the hectic morning as energy is required for the day. Once cortisol is secreted, levels of blood sugar increase as well.

Melatonin and cortisol work in contrast with each other; when one is high, the other is low. Thus, it's no surprise that melatonin levels are low and cortisol levels are high in type 2 diabetics. In addition, cortisol levels would be high in obesity.

Increase in cortisol as a result of psychological stress also paves the way for diseases. During times of stress, the blood sugar levels rise, insulin becomes desensitized, and more fat gets stored. Originally, stress is a code that was written in our genes back in the day to alert us to run from an approaching lion or predator. But now, chronic stress, which is a part of our daily lives, causes cortisol to be secreted.

If there is cortisol in the picture, blood sugar levels deteriorate. Where there is elevated cortisol, melatonin levels are low. This is how sleep deprivation at night causes chronic stress. Cortisol should be secreted during the day and melatonin at night. In every incident that these hormones deteriorate, the potential to gain weight increases. For melatonin, the ideal condition is when blood sugar is low, which is when you're hungry and in a dark environment. Only then can it overcome cortisol. It is secreted around 9:00 p.m. and peaks at 11:00 p.m., and then lasts throughout the night. For healthy functioning melatonin, the activities of blood sugar and insulin should stop before melatonin is secreted. This is why we should finish eating at least three to four hours before 9:00 p.m.

I have tried to explain the benefits of fasting, especially nighttime fasting, to our health by outlining how these hormones function. If melatonin and cortisol are the main internal circadian clock tuners, then the ideal secretion time of these hormones should not be disrupted.

In addition to melatonin, other hormones secreted at night are also circadian. The growth hormone is at the top of the list. An anabolic hormone, the growth hormone is secreted at night during sleep. It is required to keep muscles healthy. As bodily fats burn during night fasting, the growth hormone tones the muscles.

Let me remind you that the most fundamental hormone regarding nutrition and weight management is leptin, which also works according to the circadian clock. So let's have a closer look at leptin. After all, we would never feel satiated without it!

Leptin Resistance and Circadian Rhythm

Leptin is the postprandial hormone. It is secreted from the fat tissue after meals. It goes to the hypothalamus and tells the brain that we are full. If there is leptin in the system and it's active, we get the feeling of fullness.

The ghrelin hormone is leptin's antagonist. If the stomach is empty, ghrelin makes it growl—it says, "I'm hungry." When it is full, the stomach wall stretches and ghrelin goes silent. We should prefer our leptin to be dominant. If leptin is present and shows effect, then the body wouldn't ask for more food than is necessary.

So, I have just explained how leptin is secreted from fat tissues and gives the feeling of fullness. Why then do some people gain weight despite having sufficient fat tissues and leptin? Why would they still have difficulty in feeling full? The answer is hidden in the concept of "leptin resistance," which is similar to insulin resistance. Although leptin is sufficiently present, cells are not sensitive enough to perceive them as signals of satiation. As with insulin, leptin affects cells through its receptors; and in these cells, there might be a complacency towards the leptin receptors. In this case, just like it happens in insulin resistance, reaction to leptin has decreased.

As high levels of leptin create problems for overweight people, the lack of it is also an issue. Leptin deficiency causes a hormonal disorder with those who follow an entirely fat-free diet, have no body fat, lose weight very quickly, or excessively work out. Moreover, especially in women, it disrupts the menstrual cycle, which may possibly lead to infertility.

Now, let's have a look at leptin's circadian secretion:

- The best time for leptin secretion is between 2:00-4:00 a.m. This is when the growth hormone is secreted during sleep, when we are hungry enough, and hence when no insulin is present.
- If we go to bed hungry at around 11:00 p.m., which is suitable for the circadian rhythm, the system begins to burn fat while we're asleep. This burns the stored fat, especially the unwanted fat surrounding the organs.
- Just as if we have eaten fatty foods and are thus feeling full, the burning of fat in the mitochondria increases levels of leptin. If every night this were to take place, leptin insensitivity would decrease. Furthermore, insulin insensitivity would decrease. Thus, when we wake up in the morning for breakfast, our bodies would be in the right mode for burning fat, due to the previous night.

In the circadian cycle that begins with the presence of melatonin during the night, more significant biological events than those concerning body weight and insulin take place. The night segment of the circadian rhythm is the actual time to renew, regenerate, repair, and detoxify. All our decrepit cells are identified and cleaned at night. Therefore, we wake up with strong, fresh cells each morning.

Nighttime cleaning is the most crucial job performed by the metabolism. For instance, wouldn't a car that has been on the road for one hundred years need some maintenance? And, so it is with our cells. In fact, they perform this willingly. The cell that is not effective in doing its job, one which is old and worn, self-destructs. This is called apoptosis.

Voluntary Suicide Team

We call the voluntary suicide of damaged cells apoptosis.

In a healthy body, apoptosis is best undertaken in the dark at night, when melatonin is secreted and when we are hungry. Apoptosis occurs at night, when it's time for repair; it is the determination and annihilation of damaged cells that get time-worn throughout the day. Apoptosis takes place in a planned manner, usually on a daily basis. Millions of cells undergo apoptosis every day. It is crucial that this number stays within the normal range. If the number of damaged cells exceed, apoptosis may increase or cells that need to undergo apoptosis may get away. It is important that apoptosis is on target and in proportion.

If you go to bed on an empty stomach rather than a full one, apoptosis would function effectively while you sleep at night. No decrepit cells would escape, and a complete cleansing would take place.

Yes, at first glance, it may seem as if though apoptosis is something good, as we would want those bad cells to be disposed of. However, it might create a problem for some organs as the number of cells getting damaged increases before the expected lifespans of those cells are fulfilled. For example, when brain and nerve cells are destroyed through apoptosis, they wouldn't be replaced with new ones. The brain would try to perform the same functions with the decreasing number of cells happening over time. The cells that decrease in number with old age would cause shrinking of the brain, which we call atrophy. Atrophy in the brain is a condition seen in almost every elderly brain. It is a type of degeneration that is observed at advanced levels, especially in diseases such as dementia, Alzheimer's, and Parkinsons. (Einstein's brain was examined by pathologists years later; despite his old age, he showed not a single trace of atrophy—this still astonishes scientists today. Thus, intelligence and atrophy are inversely correlated.)

We can also attribute this occurrence to the atrophy in the muscles that appear with old age. This is called sarcopenia. Aging, in any case, occurs with the declining number of cells. What is important is that the cell does not become diseased before its time and is therefore not prematurely eradicated by apoptosis.

The initial answer to the question of why the cell becomes diseased before its time is free radical damage of the cell. **The primary source of free radicals within our bodies is that which is responsible for our energy production—the mitochondria, our energy powerhouses.**

The functions of mitochondria are also bound up with the circadian rhythm. When we learn how mitochondria cause more free radicals as a result of what we eat and when we eat, we will have a better understanding of the correlation between the shortened lives of cells and our own shortened lives. This is such an intricate and interconnected topic, that seeing nutrition only as a matter of weight management in this day and age is an utterly shallow approach.

Let me summarize what we essentially need to know so far: if we pronounce statements such as "since I do not gain weight, I can eat at night," we will cause cells to commit suicide before their time and cause the ideal number of cells to gradually decrease.

Let's say the life span of a liver cell is three months under ideal circumstances. If we overload it; in other words, if we burden it with toxins, stress, unnecessary intake of medicine, alcohol, and the like, this will be a further burden added during the detoxification process of each cell. As a consequence of these external toxic agents, there will be many free radicals to clean up at the micro level. Furthermore, imagine overeating in the evenings, to the point where you feel you are about to burst. We would be adding extra strain to the internal free-radical buildup in the liver cells. Thus, more cells than usual would be damaged and have to undergo apoptosis; as a result, the life of liver cells, and eventually the life of the liver itself, would be shortened. Even an organ as sturdy as the liver, which can function with the remaining twenty percent in the event that eighty percent is damaged, has a lifespan. These *accelerated cycles,* which continuously dispose of decrepit cells through apoptosis and replace them with new ones, are not desired for any of our organs. This implies that we would be utilizing the relevant cell and organ for a shorter period of time. Cell cycles also need to be at an ideal pace, as with circadian cycles.

However, sometimes there is not an exact signal for apoptosis. In other words, if there is a sudden and excessive damage to the cell—for instance, if there is a sudden and substantial free radical damage that occurs (such as trauma, oxygen deficiency due to a disruption in the blood flow, toxins, or infection), instead of the planned eradication process of apoptosis, the unplanned destruction process of necrosis would be necessary in order to deal with this overburdening situation.

Necrosis is not planned. Clearing the residues of

necrosis is much more difficult than clearing the residues of apoptosis. Apparently, when we are ill or facing trauma, more than apoptosis alone occurs in our bodies. Sudden and substantial free radical damage will cause rapid cell loss and necrosis in the tissues, leaving behind enormous amounts of waste to clean up. These cleaning and healing processes have a high price though. For example, after a heart attack, it takes three weeks to heal as we wait for the heart muscle cells in necrosis to be cleansed and new cells to be generated.

Now, somewhere in between, there is a state called necroptosis, which is neither apoptosis nor necrosis. This is mostly seen in chronic disease. It advances consistently and insidiously, and causes inflammation in the relevant areas. The reason for this is that although the body wants to clean it up, the signals received are not exactly those of apoptosis. The cells develop incompetence and are unable to receive the signals. This is usually what happens in chronic inflammatory diseases. It might occur as the result of various internal and external factors (including nutrition) or as the result of genetic inclination. If this state between apoptosis and necrosis continues long enough, it may cause transfiguration—namely, differentiation in the cells. One step further is proliferation, which is augmentation. Cystic conditions, polyps, and what is defined as benign growth are all proliferation. You already know that when it is malignant growth, we call it cancer!

My purpose in this chapter was to highlight the following: apoptosis is good, and we need to leave our bodies alone at night as well as while we're sleeping. For the body will perform its own *check-up*, while apoptosis occurring at excessive rates and amounts will be prevented. We especially need to avoid consuming "cheap fuel" such as baked goods and sweets in the evenings, as this will disrupt the *check-up* function, and cause the system to make mistakes and shift towards necropitosis instead of apoptosis. Thus, causing chronic disease to follow suit.

People do not realize how fast they age when they obstruct their circadian cycle by eating or sleeping late at night. Since we wouldn't be utilizing the apoptosis system on nights like these, disposal of worn-out cells would be prevented, causing us to be weak in our resistance against diseases and aging. We would not benefit from the night nor our sleep. Furthermore, our longevity genes would not be activated even though they are capable of being activated on a nightly basis.

When we are hungry and sleeping, in addition to the cellular cleaning system of apoptosis, the cellular recycling and spare-parts system come into operation; in other words, autophagy and mitophagy.

The Recycling System

Besides apoptosis—the suicide of the entire cell because it's damaged—a system in which decrepit cells are used by healthy cells as spare parts is active during night fasting. The 2016 Nobel Prize provides evidence for the significance of this system.

The 2016 Nobel Prize and Autophagy—Self-Devouring Cells

Not long ago, only two and a half years ago, the topic of the Nobel Prize given to the Japanese scientist Yoshinori Ohsumi was the mechanisms that use decrepit cells as spare parts.

Autophagy is a word derived from the Greek words *auto* (self) and *phagein* (eating). It simply means self-devouring. It's a mechanism that's been analyzed since the 1960s. Yet, by receiving the Nobel in 2016, this study caused a *paradigm shift* in what we knew regarding autophagy. It showed that autophagy is not only good for devouring obsolete parts but also beneficial for health through various mechanisms.

In order to acquire the energy and spare parts, autophagy primarily becomes active during hunger. According to studies, the biggest benefit of fasting is to make spare parts from obsolete cells for the process of autophagy. The mechanism of autophagy is also a mechanism for survival. It simply provides fuel by transforming the most damaged cells into energy, which is required for crucial functions.

Structural materials required for fundamental organ cells are provided by semi-damaged, old cells. In other words, spare parts are obtained from poor cells!

Isn't that a marvelous system. Studies show that the autophagy mechanism determines what is to be recycled and what is to be destroyed. Indeed, the transformation of a baby from an embryo is the product of this same mechanism. It determines which cells go, and which cells grow.

The insufficient functioning of autophagy can have many health-related consequences from neurological diseases to cancer. For instance, it has been determined that systems fighting infections get support from autophagy, as the mechanism can annihilate invasive bacteria and viruses.

Also, autophagy controls the rate of which we age through the renewal of aged cells, so they may be utilized for a more useful purpose. Autophagy that has broken down—i.e., that's not working—has a role in various diseases from widespread ones such as type 2 diabetes to other age-related diseases, as well as cancer. There are many studies on autophagy dysfunction and its relation to impotence and cancer.

There are several profound research studies being carried out that are centered on discovering the drug to regulate autophagy. That alone might be enough to give you some idea regarding the importance of autophagy. On whichever area the big pharmaceutical companies focus indicates that there's something quite significant to be found there. However, there is no need to be dismayed, as by reading this book, you will learn how to manage your own autophagy mechanism; you will not have to wait for those companies to invent a drug.

While autophagy is the reutilization of an entire cell as a spare part, mitophagy is the reutilization of the damaged mitochondria as a spare part—by other mitochondria. Both occur during nighttime nutrient starvation. In other words, when we are not eating, they are eating each other!

By means of mitophagy, autophagy, and apoptosis, nighttime nutrient starvation provides many great benefits. Now, let's have a look at the benefits of nighttime nutrient starvation.

The Benefits of the Night and Nighttime Nutrient Starvation

Nighttime nutrient starvation ensures that the brain is conserved and enhances its regeneration. The brain is the most susceptible organ against free radical damage. Our brain, which consumes a large amount of the energy produced in the body, uses stored resources to produce energy during nutrient starvation. It does this instead of using the unhealthy food we may be putting in our bodies; therefore, it works with relatively cleaner energy. As a result, if there is clean fuel, mitochondria energy production will generate less free radicals.

The free radicals' favorite spot to attack is the brain's fatty cell membrane. The poorly fed mitochondria that feed on the unhealthy nutrients we ingest during the day produce many free radicals. Via mitophagy, these bad mitochondria are overcome and used for energy during nighttime nutrient starvation. We then wake up in the morning to healthy and effective mitochondria.

Nighttime nutrient starvation is required for a healthy, durable brain. Another piece of new information we discovered in recent years is that the brain chemical BDNF escalates when we are hungry and enhances the number of mitochondria during nighttime nutrient starvation. The amount of healthy, fresh mitochondria we have is in proportion with the entire capacity of the brain. It was discovered that in comparison to rats eating constantly, rats that are hungry at night have higher levels of intelligence and learning capacity. Thus, it appears that nighttime nutrient starvation increases the capacity of the brain as well. What exercise does to mitochondria in the brain, so does nighttime nutrient starvation—it multiplies their numbers. Therefore, if we remain hungry for long periods of time, such as from evening till morning, we will benefit from this workout on our brains, as with rats.

The immune system is regulated during nighttime nutrient starvation. Immune cells called T cells get reprogrammed, and autoimmune reactions decrease. It seems that when we are hungry, old T cells are replaced with new T cells, and immune system cells such as lymphocytes and leukocytes are renewed.

Some studies about nutrient starvation show that

unwanted autoimmune attacks in the blood decrease. For instance, recovery from a stroke is faster through nighttime nutrient starvation, And in cancer, tumor cells' resistance to chemotherapy drugs decrease. Consequentially, cancer patients are recommended to fast for a couple of days before their chemotherapy sessions. However, healthy cells protect themselves against these drugs more easily. Based on research undertaken on rats, the progress of skin cancer and breast cancer is also hindered by nutrient starvation.

During nutrient starvation and nighttime nutrient starvation, the effects of insulin in the liver over the cells increase. Insulin resistance diminishes, blood sugar levels drop, glycogen—which is sugar stored in the liver—gets used up with sufficient nutrient starvation, and then fat burning takes place. Especially fat surrounding the internal organs are transformed into energy during sleep; so when we awake the proportion of our waist and hips is reduced.

During nutrient starvation, blood fats— triglycerides—are utilized for energy, and the amount of fat in the blood decreases. The heart, of course, is happy to be utilizing blood fats for energy. Moreover, cholesterol and triglyceride levels fall. It's been proven by experiments on animals that even blood pressure levels drop during nighttime nutrient starvation. **While undesirable fats are burned during nighttime**

nutrient starvation, we benefit from the most desirable aspect of burning fat, which is the moisturizing of the skin. Burning fat moisturizes the body. The process of burning fat during nutrient starvation, called beta oxidation, not only provides high levels of energy but also produces water. The water that has increased inside the cell through fat burning is different than the water we drink—it's special. It is called structured water. It means it is ready water for the body to use. The water we drink does not circulate in our bodies as it is, it is structured within our bodies. Desert animals and animals that hibernate obtain water in this way; in other words, by burning their own fat!

In nature, eating little and nighttime nutrient starvation are rewarded by a long life. When we look at the animals that live a long life, we see that their metabolisms are slow and that they are herbivores. Their constitutions generate less free radicals. Likewise, we see that fast-moving animals with fast metabolisms are carnivores, and so their constitutions produce more free radicals. As I mentioned already, we can perhaps assume that animals with a fast metabolism consume their potential life spans faster as a result of the short-term cycles of their cells. Conversely, we may go by the logic that slow-moving and less calorie-consuming herbivores such as elephants and turtles might live longer due to less input, less output, and less waste of engine-fuel.

For example, hibernation is a state that lengthens

the life expectancy; it is when no carbohydrates are consumed, no sunlight exists, and only the stored fats in the body are utilized for energy. Perhaps for animals in hibernation, time flows more slowly. Light—which indicates time, eating—which causes damage, and excessive movement are not present. This is food for thought!

Fasting throughout the night has benefits such as losing weight while sleeping, burning fat more easily the next day, overcoming insulin resistance, reducing leptin resistance, feeling full more easily. In addition to all of this, let's add the following formula as well. When we stop eating at 5 p.m., go to bed at 11 p.m., and sleep in the dark—as in compliance with our circadian rhythm—we will wake up to find that we weigh 300-500 grams less than the night before. Nighttime nutrient starvation is essential for the following: rejuvenation as old cells get burned at night, losing weight as unnecessary fats get burned, feeling full more easily the next day, and the continuation of burning fat. In a sense, the ketogenic diet also explains an aspect of this logic. But there are some shortcomings. The diet should be circadian; you shouldn't eat at night but fast.

Fasting alone is not enough, however. Personally, I do not support intermittent fasting during daytime. In our evolutionary development, there is the notion that "if there is sunlight, then we can find food;" thus, nutrient starvation during the day creates stress over the cells.

Nutrient Starvation Genes

In our two-million-year-old history, we humans always lived the same: when there was no sunlight, since it's not possible to hunt and find food, we waited in a corner—hungry. This makes total sense. For thousands of years, we couldn't find food at any time that we wanted. Being hungry for long hours at night was the usual routine for humans, as with all the other mammals. The genes were calibrated for this. If they weren't, then we wouldn't have genes called clock genes in the first place. *In conclusion, our circadian clock genes prove that both light as well as our eating habits changed how these genes work.*

Take the following as an example on this topic: in animals that were experimented on, it was found that if the circadian clock gene activation in their liver wasn't working, their genes became regulated after being left hungry for twenty-four hours.

Lab rats that were not fed for twenty-four hours in the first study, were examined in the second study while being fed for twenty-fours hours. The circadian clock genes of the lab rats that were continuously fed for twenty-four hours showed dysfunction again. In addition, these rats quickly gained weight.

In the third study, a different approach was taken. Rats were examined under the sixteen-hour-fasting and eight-hour-feeding system. In other words, they were left hungry for sixteen hours at night and given food for eight hours during the day. Once again, the rats' circadian clock genes began to function properly. They lost excess weight, did not have diabetes, and their metabolisms were regulated. The most significant detail here is this: in the third study, the rats were fed the same amount of calories in those eight hours as the ones in the second study where they were continuously fed for twenty-four hours. Nonetheless, the rats of the third study did not become ill nor gain weight. Although the same amount of calories were fed to the rats in both studies, their feeding was restricted to certain times according to the cycles of the day.

It appears that genes sensitive to food and the night are more concerned with when we eat than how much we eat. The rats who were in the *sixteen-hour-fasting and eight-hour-feeding system,* as opposed to the rats who were fed the same amount of calories over twenty-four hours, did not show any signs of the illnesses we humans suffer from with old age and malnutrition— such as diabetes, heart disease, high cholesterol, and fatty liver.

People of this era do not experience the abundance and scarcity cycles of the past, as they are continuously in the abundance mode, constantly eating, and especially eating in the evenings—which goes against the way circadian genes function. This might actually be the cause of the rise of obesity and disease rates all around the world, even more so than the consumption of processed foods.

If we add the abundance of food and the abundance of light, we are not much different than factory-farmed chickens continuously sitting under the light, constantly being fed, and forced to lay eggs with dysfunctional circadian clocks and short lives. Wouldn't you agree?

Even if we eat healthy and sleep eight hours every day, unless we follow our circadian rhythms, we cannot adequately benefit. We know that in medicine, the benefits of eating healthy and nutrient starvation are repeatedly emphasized. Thus, for people of this era, the correct explanation of the relationship between nutrition and a long, healthy life is to combine the circadian cycle with nutrient starvation.

Intermittent Fasting (IF)

I am sure that you come across the concept frequently. What is this thing called intermittent fasting—also known as IF—exactly? It can be defined as fasting from food for a certain period of time, and there are various recommendations on how to apply it.

The 5/2 Method: In this method, you eat as usual for five days, then for two days you eat very little, taking in only 500 calories. This is called the *time-restricted diet*. I've explained this diet in detail in my previous books, where I recommend restricting what you eat during the evening. I defined this as *dinner cancelling*. However, dinner-cancelling, intermittent fasting, and the time restricted diet all ultimately convey more or less the same ideas.

Eat-Stop Eat-Stop Method: In this system, you eat for twenty-four hours, and then the following twenty-four hours you eat nothing. It is a method that suggests a complete fast for two-three days of the week.

The 16/8 method: This is the most common method. You eat eight hours of the day while you fast in the remaining sixteen hours.

In light of all this information, I think the most ideal explanation could be that of the circadian-IF diet. Because, the medical justification in all these diet recommendations depends on the harmony between the circadian clock and the hours for eating. This has already been written in our genetic codes, but we are only recently taking it seriously. While long hours of fasting are recommended, not much is mentioned regarding the timing, and not much emphasis is put on it.

However, fasting that begins after 5 p.m. is the best for our circadian rhythms.

The circadian rhythm is determined by daylight and the wavelength of daylight that are perceived through the retina; thus, the most active interval of our circadian clocks is between 7:30 a.m. and 5 p.m. It is possible to consume food in a more relaxed manner within these hours. Yet... *Even if it doesn't turn dark after 5 p.m., since the wavelength of daylight is the main indicator, decreasing the amount of food intake or to completely stop it after this time is the most accurate method.*

My reasons for recommending a fast after 5 p.m. until the morning are mentioned in all the programs and interviews in which I attend, as well as in my previous books, where they are explained in detail. However, since mitochondria, which are responsible for energy production, are also circadian, I would like to add the relevant information in this book as well. Ceasing food intake according to the mitochondrial/circadian rhythm, starting at 5 p.m., increases the benefits of IF than doing it at any other time of the day. It enables us to lose weight much more easily as well.

In order to explain how mitochondria work in a circadian manner, and what would happen if we do not eat according to the circadian rhythm, we have to take a look at the biochemistry of nutrition. After all, if this book is a type of educational publication, it should not be read quickly and ought to consist of the density of information that is to be read repeatedly with underlining of essential facts. Therefore, instead of covering all topics separately and writing three different books, I preferred to combine and present to you three books' worth of information like the pieces of Lego.

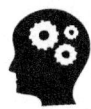

The Ultimate 5

"Food-Mitochondria-Energy"

In this chapter, I will examine the tiniest structures that function according to the circadian rhythm—micro organelles. When the subject matter is nutrition, it's impossible not to eventually speak of the mitochondria.

Since the main job of mitochondria is to provide energy, they work more passively or actively according to the pace of the metabolism and the need for energy. According to the energy requirements of the body at any given time of the day, their numbers may increase or decrease. When the energy need is lower, they go into repair mode. Studies show that with lab animals who are deflected from the daily circadian rhythm, the efficiency of the energy production of mitochondria in their bodies reduces.

The food-mitochondria-energy trio is an inseparable trio; but still, it would be a mistake to assume that we merely eat to produce energy.

Before examining the functions of mitochondria through a circadian approach, it's my priority to respond to some questions regarding nutrition.

- Why do we eat?
- How much should we eat?
- When should we eat? (I already partially responded to this.)
- How should we eat?
- What should we eat?

So, here's the Ultimate 5!

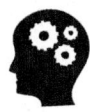

Chapter 1:

"We eat to live, not vice versa." —*Hippocrates*

In order to understand how crucial it is to eat according to our biological clock in detail, we should first figure out *why we eat*. Even a child knows that in order to live, we need to breathe and eat. But, why? Not only us but also animals, plants and bacteria eat. We cannot survive, otherwise.

A baby, that begins its journey as one cell generated by the union of two cells, feeds from its mother for nine months and ten days until it reaches approximately three kilograms. When that one tiny cell reaches three and a half kilograms, it multiplies the number of cells into trillions. Thus, our initial motivation to eat is *to provide the energy and the raw materials that enable us to grow by multiplying the number of our cells.*

How a mother eats is vital for the baby's health. Even healthy eating for nine months and ten days prevents a child from potential diseases throughout infancy, childhood, and maturing years. There are several studies on the subject matter of how the mother eats is strongly related to the child's health. Medically, there are no doubts or even differing opinions with regards to this.

What I would like to emphasize here is that it's imperative for us to understand *why we eat* and have been eating since the beginning of our lives as one-celled beings. Thus, the topic of nutrition concerns the living being before it is even born.

Experiments on lab animals have presented rather striking results. For example, a study on rats proved that unhealthy feeding throughout the period of pregnancy not only affects the offspring but also the grandchildren, who also carry certain health risks. However, when the opposite is implemented, in other words, when a rat eating unhealthy under normal circumstances eats healthy throughout its pregnancy, both the offspring and grandchildren do not have many of the health risks the mother does. These studies present impressive outcomes. It makes us think that eating healthy is probably the greatest gift our mothers can give us. (Of course, another great gift from the mother is healthy mitochondria!)

When we grow out of infancy and childhood and reach adulthood, we are obliged to eat healthy, on our own behalf. *We eat to grow. Now, in our adulthood, we feed to preserve the balance of our bodies. This balance is called homeostasis.* Homeostasis, in other words consuming nutritional raw materials agreeable to our biological structures to obtain an ideal balance, is what we call nourishment. We want balance to be on the side of our health.

Essentially, the purpose of all the cells in the body is to provide a healthy balance as long as possible. When we get injured, our body seeks to heal immediately. If we get an infection, our immune system desires to get rid of it as soon as possible. We obtain all the required nutritional raw materials and energy from of our food for thinking, moving around, and even sleeping. So then, what does it mean if we feel deprived of energy and exhausted although we eat three meals a day? Perhaps we really don't know why we eat. Because if we did know, we would provide that energy through our nutritional choices.

If you are the sort of person who connects illnesses increasing over the years to faith, genetics, and bad luck, instead of questioning your fatigue, then it means you don't know why you eat. *Despite all the existing data, if you still cannot grasp the fact that the greatest power you have against the deterioration caused by aging and for reducing diseases are related to you awareness of what you put in your mouth, then you do not know why you eat.*

The human body is a powerful biological machine. It consists of billons of cells and tens of organs; it is a biological machine designed to be perfect. This biological machine would like to work with minimum energy, maximum efficiency, and minimum waste. This simple logic is the desired performance in any machinery. And that's where the secret lies. Let me highlight the following once more: an ideal machine works with the principle of the least fuel, the highest efficiency, the least waste, the least deterioration, and the longest life. It is the same with the machine that is the human body. If each of us was a machine, we would be plugged into a wall and would obtain impeccable energy from electricity. But, we are not. So, how is this superior machine, the human body, to work flawlessly?

Our electricity is our food. That's how we obtain our energy. Each bite we take goes a long way, through hundreds of complex processes, and finally arrives at our energy factories where it is converted into energy. The function of these energy centers that we call the mitochondria is to bring out the energy found inside our food, which has been digested and has become molecular, by further breaking them down.

The actual biological end of every statement we make about food is the mitochondria. Actually, *the real answer to why we eat is to feed our mitochondria. We need to eat in a way that would increase the performance of our energy machines, which is our mitochondria.* This is a basic biological rule, and there are no exceptions to it. If we do not accept this without dispute, we'd be underestimating the importance of this matter. However, the following statement, "we should feed our mitochondria," defines our power over diseases, over aging, and even over cancer. If you want to claim, "I have the power," keep reading for further details.

Mitochondria

What is this thing called mitochondria that we can't stop talking about? Let's have a closer look...

Every cell has mitochondria.

- There may be hundreds or thousands of mitochondria in each cell.
- As the cell's need for energy increases, so does the number of mitochondria.
- The muscles, the brain, the liver, and the heart all have cells rich in mitochondria as these organs require more energy.

Mitochondria are inherited only from the mother.

- Mitochondria are not inherited from the father.
- Everyone comes from a long line of mitochondria inherited from the women in their families—from their mothers, their paternal and maternal grandmothers, and in this way, from a similar mitochondrial generation of their oldest female ancestor—and passes on the mitochondria to following generations.

The symbiosis approach, which claims that the ancestors

of mitochondria are one-celled bacteria, is generally acknowledged. The physical structure of mitochondria shows similar aspects to one-celled bacteria.

Mitochondria Have Their Own DNA.

They are portrayed as mtDNA. The presence of mito-DNA is the reason for humans' extraordinary aspects. Although it should be given as much importance as our main DNA, it's been kept in the background until only recently. When we are searching for causes of diseases, the first place to look is not our main DNA as we commonly know it, but the mito-DNA. Recent studies on mito-DNA indicate how a more accurate explanation is required with regards to diseases including cancer that are unexplainable through genetics. And all of this brings one question to mind: could scientists have been looking at the wrong DNA all this time? I believe they have.

Whether the mitochondria work properly or not sets the fate of all the diseases that come to mind. In light of various studies, I will list some of them below. A problem either in mitochondria or in mito-DNA has been identified in all these diseases.

Some of the Diseases Related to Mitochondria

Diabetes Type 2	Cancer
Neurodegenerative Diseases	Dementia

Cardiovascular Diseases	Muscle Loss
Muscle Weakness	Fatigue
Exercise Intolerance	Fibromyalgia
Chronic Fatigue Syndrome	Muscle Pain
Migraine	Constipation
Bowel Issues	Respiratory Disorder
Eyelid Impairment	Feeling Cold/the Chills
Hand Tremor	Eyesight Problems
Hearing Impairment	Polycystic Ovary
Obesity	Thyroid Issues
Aging of Skin	

I could continue with the list, but I don't see the point. Because, I know you already see the logic: if there is a cell, then that cell has a duty; and in order to fulfill that duty, energy is required. If there's not enough energy, then obviously the cell's work will be compromised. In short, the performance of the cells depends on the performance of their mitochondria. It is the same with organs as well. In a nutshell, at the core of it all, somehow all diseases are related to mitochondria. *If we are having a discussion on general health, it is actually the health of the mitochondria that we are discussing.*

Let's look at another characteristic of our mitochondria—one that is more striking. It is actually our mitochondria that breathe. Mitochondria cannot produce energy without oxygen. The importance of breathing is equal to the health of the mitochondria. When mitochondria do not function well, there will be hypoxia in tissues—which is the lack of oxygen. If mitochondria are not healthy, then the breath you take is, in reality, not a breath.

We damage our mitochondria as a result of our unhealthy eating habits and lifestyles. That's why the oxygen cannot be utilized efficiently in the cells. In fact, we all live in a constant state of hypoxia, constantly lacking oxygen. This is called pseudo-hypoxia. Here is the implication: we are all slowly suffocating! And, we are not even aware of it!

If we talk about bodyweight and calories, then this can again be related to how mitochondria function. Good functioning mitochondria produce good energy. If mitochondria are not functioning well, then food turns into calories instead of energy. This is what happens even if we do not eat excessively.

Looking at how obesity is a global epidemic, is it not obviously clear that we are missing something, somewhere? In medical circles, though not widespread, it is understood that the solution lies in protecting the health of our mitochondria.

All around the world, not only weight gain but also

issues on healthy living and longevity are researched with regards to mitochondria. Nearly in most diseases, the common denominator is whether mitochondria are healthy or not. In addition, new methods concerning the prevention of diseases now focus on the protection of the mitochondria. Let me give you a futuristic tip: disease treatments in the future will be undertaken with transplants of the mitochondria.

The Structure of Mitochondria:

MITOCHONDRIA

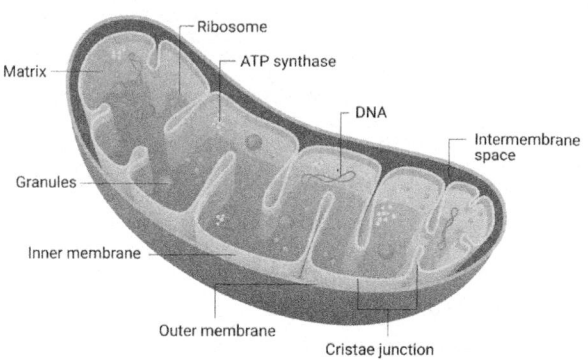

Now, let's get to know the structure of our valuable mitochondria in more detail. While we're looking for answers to the above questions as we move forward in this book, and especially trying to grasp the relations between eating habits and diseases, we need to comprehend the structure of mitochondria thoroughly since that is the area in which all takes place.

Mitochondria are organelles; in other words, they are tiny organs within cells. Whatever the organs do for our body, in a similar way, organelles are structures that operate within our cells. Mitochondria are surrounded with two layers of membrane: the inner membrane and the outer membrane. The inner membrane of mitochondria is highly folded—just like the folded surface of the intestines or the brain. In the human body, these folds are utilized in order to expand the surface area of highly functioning areas. Due to the folds of the inner membrane, where energy production takes place, mitochondria may have a wide surface area. As a result of the folds, the area to produce energy is multiplied. This is similar to the projections, namely villus, on the surface of intestines that create more space in order to absorb nutrients. This is also similar to the folds of the brain; as the folds on the brain's surface multiply, we become creatures with highly developed and greater functioning brains.

I would like to emphasize this folded structure for the following reasons. As with the *leaky gut condition* that develops when the folds of the intestines are punctured, if the folds of mitochondria become damaged, likewise, a leaky mitochondria condition follows. This is actually the starting point of many diseases. I will be discussing this further in the upcoming pages.

Aside from the inner and outer membrane of the mitochondrion, there is the space within the inner membrane. This space is called the matrix. I believe you'll find it rather easy to remember the word *matrix*. As you may remember, there was a film by the same name. There's the *blue pill, red pill...* For now, let's just keep in mind that the matrix we are talking about here is in the depths of the mitochondrion, and it has a role to play in energy production.

Energy Production in Mitochondria:

Ninety percent of the energy supply of the entire the body is provided by mitochondria, which are the final destination for nutrients. Mitochondria are the digestive systems in the cell. They obtain nutrients at their final stage and garner their subatomic energy. We can consider them as a sort of oven—burning food with oxygen and extracting energy and heat from them. We call this process, since oxygen is involved, cellular respiration. In other words, mitochondria are also the lungs of the cell.

Cellular respiration is the process of oxygen and nutrients entering the mitochondria and transforming into energy. If we cannot survive for more than three to four minutes without breathing, then we need to understand the following: if we don't have the required oxygen, no energy will be generated in the mitochondria. Therefore, if our mitochondria do not function, we will die in three minutes. In the movies, the moment the zigzag heart beat line on the monitor turns into a flatline, it is the moment when mitochondria of the heart cannot produce energy, the heart muscles cannot pump blood because of the lack of energy, and the heart stops beating. Now that I've got your attention on the energy production of mitochondria in such a dramatic manner, I hope you are more curious about learning some more biochemical details about it.

Mitochondria are tiny organelles, yet they have a hard-working capacity. Although they are tiny structures, you may think of them as power centers. Mitochondria have odd habits. For example, in order to produce energy, they have preferences among nutrients. Mitochondria produce energy from all three main food groups—glucose, fat, and protein. However, their order of preference is as follows: first, glucose; second, fats; and then, proteins. **Glucose is prioritized because it is fuel that burns easily**. Have a look at your plate. Food that can easily transform into glucose is the cheapest fuel. The others come into play only if there is no glucose or the amount is insufficient.

Nonetheless, glucose being the first choice brings many problems with it. Glucose is actually *dirty cheap fuel!* The rest of this book is dedicated to explaining how problems occur as a result of using this fuel.

When there is no or very little glucose, breaking down the second choice—fats—is something healthy cells do very easily. Cells that can quickly make the *metabolic switch* between breaking down glucose or fat as required are the healthiest cells. A healthy cell should immediately be able to make this metabolic switch as needed. This metabolic switch gets really difficult to manage as we get older, when we mostly feed on glucose, or when a health condition is present. In cancer, there is almost no switch. The cancer cell prefers not to make the metabolic shift. Glucose has first rank and proteins have second in nutrient preference, but fats never have rank. They cannot. I will tell you why…

In every chapter of this book, you will read about the nutrient preferences of mitochondria in detail. But for now, let's have a look at why glucose is the first choice and how it transforms into the chemical energy called ATP.

Let me proceed with the simplest explanation. Imagine this is a film. Now, fast forward the digestion stages to the scene where glucose knocks on the cell's door and begin right there. This is the moment after we eat when glucose is digested and transferred to our blood, and arrives at the door of the cell through the circulatory system.

Depending on the level of glucose in the blood, the insulin hormone that is secreted from the pancreas introduces glucose into the cell. This is not always possible, however. In the case when glucose is unable to get inside, it generates what we call diabetes and insulin resistance. In order for you to better comprehend these diseases caused by glucose being the first choice, I will continue explaining what happens when the cell is still healthy. Insulin invites glucose inside. And, this is where our film begins.

Glycolysis: Glucose's First Major Event

In the first scene, glucose is processed in the first part of the cell identified as cytoplasm (not the mitochondrion—don't get confused). The process occurs in the following way as stated below.

From glucose *pyruvate* is formed. In this phase, two units of ATP are gained. The film has started, and we have already met with our next actor after glucose—pyruvate.

The name of this process is glycolysis.

We Must Remember Glycolysis. Why?

1. It produces two units of ATP, which is *very little* energy.
2. It is an energy substitute that has *short-term* use in case mitochondria cannot be used.
3. In cancer or chronic diseases, its *long-term* use is actually the cause of these diseases. (Yes, cancerous cells always prefer to use glycolysis. It doesn't prefer to take the path from glycolysis to mitochondria. On the other hand, noncancerous cells do not prefer to use glycolysis for a long time,

because less energy is produced through this process. Cells cannot perform their duty with that amount of energy. But, a cancerous cell does not perform its regular duties anyway. It just struggles not to die. That's why it prefers to use glycolysis. It is known that especially aggressive tumors use mitochondria to multiply instead of producing energy. This is called the *Warburg effect*. Having short-term glycolysis and continuing with the rest in the mitochondrion are essential for health.)

4. What actually matters is that, in glycolysis, there is no oxygen. It is known as *oxygen-free*, in other words, as anaerobic energy production. Glycolysis works just like fermentation, like in making pickles.

5. The only advantage of glycolysis for the body is that it is quick. The duration of glucose turning into energy through glycolysis is twenty times faster than glucose breaking down in the mitochondria in order to be transformed into energy. That's why it is suitable for cancerous cells.

Pyruvate formed by glycolysis has two paths lying

ahead, and it is supposed to pick one of the two.

Pyruvate takes the road towards mitochondria if:

- There's oxygen around.
- Mitochondria are healthy.
- Little food has been consumed.

And this is actually what we want.

Yet, not all of the pyruvate goes to the mitochondrion. Some parts remain in glycolysis. They get fermented and lactic acid is formed. This happens when:

- There's not enough oxygen.
- Mitochondria are damaged.
- Excessive amount of food is consumed (especially carbohydrates).

What Is Lactic Acid?

What do we know about lactate? Lactate—also known as lactic acid—is acid. It reduces the pH of the cells to acidic value. But, cells are supposed to have an ideal pH value. Catalyzer enzymes within the cell only work when the cell is at its ideal pH value. As lactic acid production escalates, the pH of the cell becomes acidic, which is not suitable for the cell. It's necessary for lactate to be expelled from the cell, after which the liver tries to clean. (Since cancerous cells insist on glycolysis, they produce excessive amounts of lactic acid. And in order not to die, they remove that lactic acid from the cell. It gets very acidic outside of the cell. So much so that you can forget that the immune system has difficulty in determining the cancerous cell; because, even chemotherapy drugs have a difficult time approaching the cancerous cell due to the *acidic coat*.)

Events Taking Place in the Mitochondria

Let's return to our ideal cell and to our movie's main theme, the mitochondria. Let the pyruvate go to the mitochondria.

Pyruvate coming from glycolysis first enters the matrix inside mitochondria and goes into a constantly circulating chain—the TCA cycle. In the *TCA cycle* (it is called a cycle due to its constant circulation), byproducts are generated from the pyruvate. The most important byproducts are NADH and FADH2, which are the final molecular phase of nutrients.

NAD already exists in the TCA cycle. When you add an H, it becomes NADH.
NAD+H=NADH
Similarly, FAD also exists, and an H is added as well.
FAD+2H=FADH2

You may wonder where this H, which we add to the existing values, comes from. H comes from nutrients. *The final phase of the energy inside the morsels we put in*

our mouths is the electron within hydrogen, which is
represented here with an H.

Hydrogen in NADH and FADH2 is the part that
actually forms the energy. These two molecules are
electron carriers. Every nutrient, no matter what we eat,
will turn into these eventually. The difference between
the two is:

All carbohydrates turn into NADH.
All fats turn into FADH2.

The film at this point takes a turn towards the surreal,
which wouldn't have you longing for sci-fi films, as it
continues with the dispute between electrons and
protons inside the hydrogen atom.

Abundant Atom of the Universe: Hydrogen

Hydrogen is the simplest atom. It has one proton and
one electron. The richest, lightest, and simplest atom
on the earth, hydrogen carries inside itself the energy
that comes from food.

Up until this point, I have broken down glucose.
And now I will do the same for hydrogen. Yes,
producing energy is exactly that—breaking down the
atom. It is a huge task. After NADH and FADH2 are
formed, we move on to the inner membrane from
mitochondria's matrix. Now, we are on mitochondria's
inner membrane.

Mitochondria Inner Membrane

We are on the inner membrane with folds, which I mentioned at the beginning. In order to explain the significance of this folded membrane, it wouldn't be enough even if I write my sentences in bold capital letters, highlight them, and punctuate with an exclamation point. That's why I will tell you straightforwardly. The mitochondria inner membrane is the most important part of the body. If the path to immortality were to be discovered some day, I believe the answer would lie here.

On this inner membrane of the mitochondria, there is the **electron transport chain** (ETC). This is where high amounts of energy is actually generated. All the energy obtained until now has been in modest amounts. As you can understand by looking at the name of the chain, the electron transport chain is where nutrient electrons are utilized. Its name is not glucose transport chain nor fat transport chain nor protein transport chain; it is electron transport chain. The feature we most seek after in food is related to the electrons coming here.

The ETC is also called the respiration chain; the most important metabolic action in our body takes place here. Let's get acquainted with this chain.

Complex Chain: The ETC

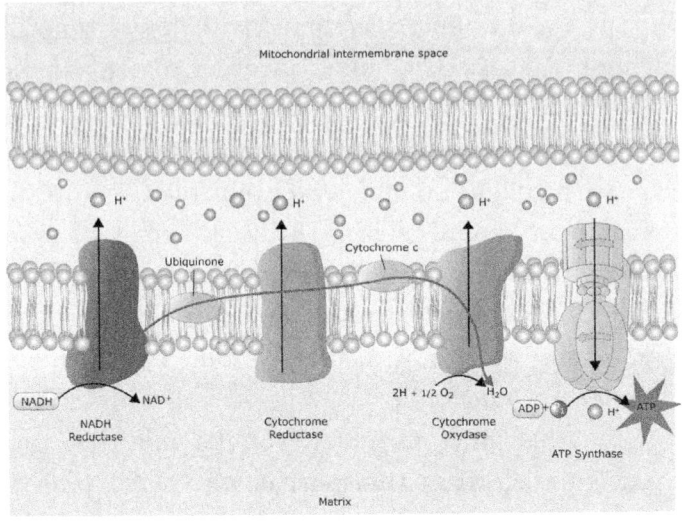

The ETC, which is the respiration chain, is where food is transformed into high amounts of ATP. So that the ETC can multiply, the mitochondria membrane's surface area was expanded with the help of its folded structure. Therefore, a high amount of ETC can settle on it, and a marvelous energy production area may be generated. If we compare the energy produced here per square meter to the energy produced on the sun, the ETC energy produced here per unit is much more. All ETCs constantly produce energy as strong as lightning.

If we make an analogy of the ETC to a train, it would have five stations:

- Stations 1, 2, 3, 4, and 5. We call these

Complexes. Complex 1, 2, 3, 4, and 5. The purpose of these stations is to reveal the energy inside electrons that are carried in by nutrients. They accomplish their tasks one by one. Electrons coming from nutrients flow between stations 1 and 4. Electrons consecutively move from one station to the other, one at a time, and with a certain speed. An electron should not arrive at the station before the previous one leaves. Proper flow and the speed of the flow between stations are vital.

- Electron flow stops at the fourth station. ATP is formed at the final station—Complex 5.
- Regarding nutrition and diseases, Complex 1 is the one we are most concerned about.
- Complex 1, which is the first station, is where NADH-carrying electrons coming from glucose enters.
- There's a rule: electrons coming from carbohydrates always enter Complex 1 via NADH.
- NADH leaves its H at Complex 1 and transforms into NAD again.
- Transformation between NADH/NAD should take place at a certain pace.

- H Hydrogen's journey begins at the ETC. The electron inside H hydrogen is signified with a minus (-). The proton is indicated with a plus (+). The entire story behind this energy production is based on the positive and negative parts' separating from each other.

Starting at Complex 1, these electrons move through Complexes 2, 3, and 4, leaving behind the energy they have inside. The energy is in the electrons. And at Complex 4 waits the oxygen we inhale. This is where oxygen comes into the picture. The unification of oxygen with electrons turns into water at Complex 4. Everything I have explained until now has been the experience of hydrogen's negative (-) electrons.

In addition, there are the positive (+) protons of hydrogen. What happened to them? As electrons flow from Complexes 1 through 4, the energy generated is utilized to push the protons of hydrogen through the inner membrane to the other side. Hence, as the electrons of hydrogen stay on the membrane and flow from one Complex to the other, the protons of hydrogen are pushed to the other side of the membrane with the energy provided from the electron-flow.

Normally, since the inner membrane of the mitochondria—where this all takes place—is not permeable, it can only be pushed to the other side by the energy of electrons. There would therefore be positives on one side and negatives on the other side of the membrane. This difference, the (+) and (-) electric difference of two sides, creates voltage. It is a simple rule that if on each side of the membrane that is not permeable there is ion intensity, then there is electrical disparity. We call this *gradient*. This negative and positive disparity generates a voltage gradient on the membrane. Essentially, a battery is generated, in the simplest sense. An electric voltage is generated on the membrane.

Battery Charge and ATP

We could say this process is much the same with what happens when we fill a dam with water. As with the pressure that forms on the wall of the dam, some sort of voltage forms on the membrane. Analogous to obtaining electricity out of that water dam and releasing the accumulated water, those protons are allowed to come back through Complex 5 in a controlled manner. At Complex 5, as with the water flowing channel in the dam, there's an engine called ATP that enables passage. Protons putting pressure outside of the membrane flow over this engine like a waterfall. The power of this flow enables the activity of the ATP engine. And with this, our basic energy unit ATP is generated.

Providing energy in the electron transport chain inside mitochondria's inner membrane is actually quite comparable to the functioning of a hydroelectric terminal. ATP is our energy unit. We struggle with all the stuff of eating, digesting, and the like, to produce ATP. It is short for adenosine triphosphate; it withholds energy in the phosphate, which is indicated with the letter P. If energy is required, these three phosphates are used up as two phosphates or one phosphate for all the functions of the body. As phosphates decrease, the names change: ATP (three—3 phosphates), ADP (duo—two phosphates), AMP (mono—one phosphate).

ATP produced in this way is used for the immense amount of energy that the body needs to function. As for the amount of ATP, it is a means of communication for the entire body. To understand if there's energy in the body, look at the amount of ATP, as it's a determinant for the metabolism. Whether it is required to break down fat or store it is determined by the proportions of ATP-ADP-AMP. This is just like a battery!

When ATP is plenty, the battery is fully charged. When ADP is plenty, then three quarters of it is full. When AMP is plenty, it means that the battery is almost empty.

The level at which the battery is charged affects the circadian clock as well. It even affects sleep. This seems very simple, right? When the battery is empty, we feel sleepy. Actually, it's not that simple; but, I'll talk about that a bit further down the road.

Yes, every time the ATP engine at station 5

revolves, it adds a phosphate to the molecule ADP and turns it into ATP. Ultimately, the energy of nutrients gets placed in phosphate, indicated as P, and nutrients are transformed into chemical energy.

ADP+P=ATP (generation of energy; added phosphate)
ATP=ADP+P+ ENERGY (consumption of energy; consumed phosphate)

The ATP engine constantly revolves, and ADP quickly transforms into ATP. ATP should quickly transform back into ADP, because the minute ATP is formed, energy is ready and should be used immediately. ATP cannot accumulate. Once ATP is produced, it should be used right away and convert back into ADP from ATP. *ATP cannot accumulate.*

Since we need excessive amounts of energy, this cycle continues to function at an unbelievable pace. The body needs so much energy for daily errands that it produces ATP per day as much as its weight. For example, if you weigh 80 kilograms, then you produce 80 kilograms of ATP. Yet, if ATP cannot be accumulated, then how can 80 kilograms of it be produced? It is because there's a constant cycle. It is generated, broken down, and then generated again. The cessation of this cycle is not in congruence with life. ATP production entirely stops at the time of death. Wouldn't it be wonderful if we had ATP reserves?

A Rule: ATP cannot be stored. This is where the problems begin.

What about us? What happens when:

- We continue to eat even if there is no need for energy?
- We continue to eat even if we are not going to use ATP?

Since ATP cannot be stored and needs to be consumed as soon as it is produced, even if we produce extra ATP, its production will stop if it's not used. This is the system. ATP decreases, ADP increases. The ADP/ATP cycle breaks down.

A Rule: ADP and ATP should always be transformed into each other at a certain level.

Let's identify these metabolic events that should occur as *flow*, or *cycle*. "Stopping" here is not in congruence with life. If something is amiss with these cycles, it is the reason we become ill.

We will learn about the cost of disrupting cycles by unhealthy or excessive eating, and by not living according to our biorhythm. But before the excessive parts, let's continue to learn about the normal parts.

How Much ATP Is Normally Produced?

Not that we understand what ATP production is all about, let's take a look at the amount of ATP. If we return to our first actor, glucose, we will remember that we had obtained two ATPs through glucose. But, if pyruvate provided by glycolysis gets into the mitochondria, it produces thirty-six more ATPs.

If there were no mitochondria, we would have been confined to two ATPs. But now that we have mitochondria, we can produce thirty-six more ATPs with the same raw material. Although the beginning is the same—in other words, it begins with only one glucose, the production is multiplied by fifteen.

Therefore, the implication here is that the main purpose of having mitochondria is to obtain plenty of energy from small amounts of nutrients. This is the survival instinct! Two billion years ago, when there was no oxygen on Earth, both glucose (i.e., food) and oxygen were scarce for single-celled creatures, who were obliged to utilize glucose by producing energy through fermentation without oxygen (glycolysis). However, this meant obtaining a rather low amount of energy (two ATPs), and so, they couldn't develop. Then came a bit more intelligent cells. They learned to use oxygen; and by collaborating under the same roof, they formed the first cell, after which they generated plenty of energy from small amounts of raw material. This is how turbocharged mitochondria were generated. Mitochondria later learned how to burn fat and attain ultra-plus engine power, where they were able to produce 129 ATPs from one gram of fat.

So, you have now seen that the response to the question of why we eat is much more complicated than for merely obtaining energy. We actually eat to convert little amounts of food into turbocharged energy! For this turbocharged energy, we use mitochondria. If it weren't for this, we wouldn't be complicated beings undertaking complicated functions. To summarize, mitochondria are organs that can provide turbocharged energy out of little fuel!

But what if there's too much fuel? Can mitochondria constantly generate more energy? Here is a question with an answer worth a million dollars! Unfortunately, no!

More nutrients than the speed of mitochondria can convert into fuel, choke the mitochondria, and therefore choke the engine. I say choke on purpose. *Yes, being overweight and having a chronic disease are sort of like choking.* Under these circumstances, mitochondria do not function properly. When mitochondria do not function properly, oxygen cannot be used to its full capacity; what we medically identify as low level of hypoxia—chronic lack of oxygen—goes hand in hand with all diseases. This hypoxia is only one of the consequences of eating more than necessary.

Now, here's the answer to the million-dollar question above. *To eat excessively and/or unhealthy are connected with diseases, for they disrupt the cycle of mitochondria.*

So, what disrupts the mitochondria cycle?
How much eating is excessive eating?

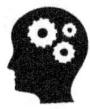

Chapter 2:

HOW MUCH SHOULD WE EAT?

There's No Such Thing as Free Food!

In order to comprehend how eating unhealthy makes us ill, first we need to understand how mitochondria get corrupted. After all, diseases start at a cellular level. The actual reason of mitochondria dysfunction is the inefficient ETCs causing more free radicals than usual while obtaining energy out of nutrients. Let me repeat that: *the actual reason of mitochondria dysfunction is the inefficient ETCs causing more free radicals than usual while obtaining energy out of nutrients.*

I had previously mentioned that ETCs are on the mitochondria inner membrane. They consist of 5 complexes. With the help of oxygen, they burn nutrient electrons. By the power of electrons, they send protons to the gap between membranes. Protons are thrown beyond membranes by Complexes 1, 3 and 4. And then flowing like a waterfall over the 5th Complex, they generate energy. So far so good.

Now, let's discuss the problems regarding energy production.

The Price of Energy: No Food Is for Free!

The ETC machine never performs one hundred percent. Even under the most ideal circumstances, there would be some leak—somewhere between 0.04% and 4%. The name of this leak is free radicals. However, the system can clean this up. Therefore, the increase of this leak to an amount more than the system can clean up is what causes diseases. All chronic degenerative diseases and aging develop together with the escalating amount of free radicals and dysfunctional mitochondria.

A Rule: The largest source of free radicals in the body is the ETC of mitochondria.

In order to understand the reason why more free radicals than usual are generated at the ETC as a result of malnutrition, first you must understand how they are generated under normal circumstances.

How Free Radicals Are Generated?

Under normal circumstances, free radicals are also produced in ETC complexes. *The station that produces the most free radicals is the first station, Complex 1. This station generates the most free radicals. Unfortunately, Complex 1 is the most common route. Most carbohydrates use this route. Especially after consuming simple carbohydrates, this route gets real busy.*

Complex 3 generates less free radicals compared to Complex 1.

Complex 2 does not generate free radicals. It's a small complex. Its purpose is to provide extra electrons. If we do not eat any carbohydrates, fat enters the system through this place, and gets converted into energy. If there are no carbohydrates around, and if there's nutrient starvation, the body uses this route to burn the stored fat. At this point, we can figure out how free radical generation decreases during nutrient starvation.

If the electron flow through the complexes is not fluent and at the right pace, free radicals will generate, as there would not be sufficient energy to push the protons to the other side of the membrane. In order to avoid this from happening, there are two supporters to carry electrons between complexes. Electrons arriving at Complex 1 and Complex 2 are carried to Complex 3 by a molecule we are all too familiar with—Coenzyme Q10.

I'm guessing that you've heard and read a lot about **Coenzyme Q10**. But the real story here is that Coenzyme Q10 carries electrons from Complexes 1 and

2 to 3 via the ETC. This is what it does. Without Coenzyme Q10 there can be no electron flow; hence, no energy can be generated. We can say that Coenzyme Q10 is the matchstick for the electron chain. It ignites everything. Electrons arriving at Complex 3 by CoQ10 are carried to Complex 4 by another carrier— **cytochrome C.**

We've heard a lot about Coenzyme Q10, but I predict we haven't heard much about cytochrome C. Yet, it has a very important function. Cytochrome C is actually a dimmer. I'm referring to the electric switches that control the lighting; they increase or decrease the amount of light. That's what a cytochrome C is—it is the switch that decreases the electron flow at the ETC when needed. *If there are more than the usual number of free radicals around, it is the switch that completely turns off the energy production.* Therefore, energy production is under very strict control at the ETC. If there is an ETC present that is producing insufficient energy, cytochrome C turns that off. By doing so, it protects the body to a certain degree.

However, there's another situation at hand. There is so much free radical leakage from the ETC due to aging Mitochondria and malnutrition that the local turning-off activity at the center can no longer solve the problem. In this case, the solution is to switch off all the cells. Hence, we continue to live with decreasing number of cells. In reality, aging is a state in which we are stuck with reduced, dysfunctional, and worn-out cells. The objective is to use the same cell for as long as possible with the highest efficiency while we are still healthy. The intelligent solution to this is to protect the ETC electric centers—in other words, the mitochondria.

Why do we feel lethargic even though we sustain ourselves and our vitality with the energy that we get through nutrients? We feel tired even after just waking up, and we spend the day dragging our bodies from one point to another with difficulty. Perhaps, you've been diagnosed with something such as chronic fatigue syndrome, burn out syndrome, or fibromyalgia? There is only one solution to this: you must reinforce the energy production centers!

I Can't Get Electricity!

The top perpetrator shutting down ETC stations by way of cytochrome C is overeating. When you eat more than the ATP you can use, electrons cannot convert into ATP anymore, electron flow stops, and the free radical leakage increases. In addition, cytochrome C shuts down the station. You eat but still feel tired. Then you start to question why you can't get energy from food. You're baffled when you feel sleepy after you eat. You gain weight even if you eat very little. These complaints are familiar; but, in order to figure out what you are doing wrong, you must learn the basics. That's why I will summarize everything I've explained so far.

Maybe you're feeling as if you are back in your high school chemistry class. However, this much boredom will come back to you as health and longevity! Trust me… now read the summary.

Glucose from nutrients:

- first transforms into pyruvate through glycolysis and then into the electrons in NADH in the mitochondria matrix TCA cycle;
- passes on to the ETC on the mitochondria membrane via electrons;
- makes its way to the oxygen in Complexes 1,2,3, and 4.

At the same time, with the strength gained from the electron flow, Hydrogen protons are sent to the other side of the membrane. Complex 5 is where protons flow down like a waterfall. This power of flow makes the ATP engine revolve.

Every time the ATP engine revolves, phosphate is added to ADP and ATP is generated.

Ok, that's all the reminding I will do.

Cycles and Flow of Time

This reminder was so that you could completely comprehend that everything is about flows and cycles at a certain pace. These cycles should continue at a certain pace, and never stop

TCA revolves all the time.
NAD/NADH transforms to each other constantly.
The ATP engine revolves all the time.
ADP/ATP transforms to each other all the time.
The aim of all these cycles is to keep the ETC electrons flowing steadily.

Electrons constantly flow in the ETC. If the speed of this flow slows down, we age. If it's fast and in balance, we stay young! In my opinion, even the relativity of time is hidden in this flow. If the ETC electron flow was at the speed of light, then we wouldn't have the concept of time. Wherever the speed is closer to the speed of light, that's where time slows down. If the complexes are good and strong, electrons flow very quickly via a sub-atomic method known as quantum tunneling over the ETC. If the ETC is shorter, then speed gains momentum. When the electron transport chain stretches in length (malnutrition and poor living conditions being the cause) it slows down the momentum. If the chain stretches one angstrom, then the speed slows down by ten percent. As a result, the energy production decreases and free radical production increases. In short, we age. Essentially, as the ETC slows down, we age.

Cold ice therapies that athletes apply is for shortening the length of the ETC and fastening the quantum tunneling flow of electrons. This enables regeneration and provides energy. That's why taking a cold shower after your regular shower makes you feel more energetic. In this way, functioning of the quantum world in the ETC increases. If we do not prepare the ideal setup for rules in the quantum world to function, then we pay for it as "time." All in all, matter is solidified and slowed-down light that has escaped from the quantum world due to its having slowed down.

In the microcosmic universe of the cell, all events take place as revolving or as flowing. Also, in the macrocosmic universe, everything revolves or flows. Nothing stops. Electrons inside the atom constantly revolve. Electrons constantly flow from one atom to another. Light flows, time flows, days flow, nights flow. Planets revolve, moon revolves, the earth revolves, the galaxy revolves, seasons revolve, everything flows, everything revolves. Nothing stops.

It would be wise not to meddle with cycles. As of now, protecting our night and day cycles is the smartest thing we can do. Circadian cycles are of time as well. If the cycle goes faster, the biological time goes faster, and you will reach the end very quickly. Entropy will have an early win.

What Is Entropy?

The definition of entropy is that everything in the

universe is sort of sliding into a state of disintegration, a state of breaking down. It is a universal rule that all incidents are intended to increase entropy. It is inevitable as you can see!

For living beings, this means moving towards decay and towards death. All living beings are drawn to universal entropy, towards decay. On the other hand, every living being struggles and fights against entropy. Thus, life is a battle with entropy. *The longer a living being resists entropy, the longer they live. Diseases can be cured as long as we resist entropy. Old age is the rise of inner entropy, and death is the ultimate win of entropy.*

Unfortunately, entropy always wins! All living beings die. When we talk about a healthy, long life, we talk about delaying universal entropy's victory. Living a healthy life means supporting our system that is already naturally working to fight entropy.

To fight against entropy requires energy. And providing that energy is the task of our mitochondria. The moment there is no flow or circulation of energy production, entropy wins. Thus, if the flow and circulation slows downs in mitochondria, diseases develop.

Now, let's see how the problems of flow and circulation appear in our daily lives.

The Food-Disease Connection

"There have been so many fish who, despite living confidently in the water, have succumbed to their greed and taken the bait." —Rumi

In order to live a healthy life, we need to have an existence and cycles as harmonious as the whirling dervishes. If flows and cycles are disrupted, we gain weight. We should eat in quantities that would not disrupt these flows and cycles and at the right time, so that they continue as they should.

On the other hand:

- The ETC chain should be at a certain momentum.
- Electrons should flow from Complexes 1 to 4 at a certain pace.
- Then, protons should enter the ATP engine through the gaps between

membranes at a certain momentum.

- ADP, taking in a phosphate and transforming into ATP through this engine, should be used the minute it becomes ATP and transform into ADP again. This cycle should be continuous.

What happens if ATP is not used and the cycle is disrupted, thus obstructing the ATP/ADP transformation?

ATP production stops immediately. Unfortunately, possessing extra ATP is not a possibility. If ATP is not used fast enough, the ATP engine stops. In consequence, ADP increases and ATP decreases even though ADP/ATP proportions should remain at a certain level.

We cannot solve the problem by stopping ATP formation. If we continue to eat, electrons continue to enter the ETC. Yet, they cannot be transformed into ATP.

In the end, electrons accumulate in the ETC chain.

But they cannot flow. They form a puddle behind! The energy within cannot be extracted. However, what pushes protons to the other side of the membrane is the energy we obtain from electrons. If there is no energy, protons remain on the membrane. The difference of (-) and (+) between two sides of the membrane diminishes. **The electric voltage on the membrane decreases. But, this voltage is vital.**

The logic is that if the end of the chain does not flow, then the beginning of the chain will cease as well. The TCA cycle will slow down, and pyruvate entering the TCA can no longer thrust electrons toward the mitochondria. Since there is no need for ATP, it will get stored as pyruvate triglyceride, which is fat. If there are excessive amounts of ATP and they're not used, the system will store whatever we eat.

- With this reasoning, we can see the benefit of exercise, which means the utilization of the ATP that emerges from the ETC.
- Furthermore, we also see the benefits of eating less, which means the existing amount of electrons won't choke the ETC.

Let's get back to the solution—attaining the desired weight. And I promise you, I will give you the formula for eating without gaining weight; but health is more important than beauty. First, we must understand why overeating concerns us not only with regards to weight accumulating on the hips but also the diseases it brings with it.

Overeating: At The Expense Of Your Health, Not Just Your Weight

Why do we attribute eating to diseases? Yes, I'm aware you feel as if you've been thrown into the middle of a biology or chemistry class; and, although I've been discussing this topic for pages now, you still can't make the connection. Yes, dear readers, the connection has not yet been made. So, keep reading! We will take a look at why it doesn't end at the chubby hips and bellies when we eat excessively.

First of all, let's remember once more that we are in need of and dependent on cycles and flows. Now, let's continue in more detail. *If electrons enter the ETC too quickly before Complex 1 sends its electrons to the next Complex, the newcomer clogs the flow.* Usually, only four per one thousand and four percent of the ETC flow are produced as free radicals. When the flow is clogged, the percentage of free radicals increase.

If electrons hop consecutively from Complexes 1 through 4, then there will be enough energy to push the protons through the membrane to the other side. If this does not occur, there won't be enough energy to propel the protons. It will turn into a battlefield of free radicals!

In addition, when the protons are not thrusted to the other side of the membrane, *the electric voltage of the membrane decreases.* The decrease of the membrane voltage and the swarms of free radicals hovering around cause something vital: *the disintegration of the membrane!*

Molecules that we call free radicals attack the membranes most easily. Since the ETC is on the inner membrane, free radicals first do damage in the place they were generated. They first oxidize and then break down the membrane. You do realize that the

disintegration of the mitochondria inner membrane—
which we define as impermeable, durable, and vital—
signals a terrible outcome, right? If it were possible to
create a horror film effect in a book, this would be just
the right spot to do it!

Leaky Mitochondria

Yes, this is where we need the horror movie effects. All
around the world, scientists spending a lifetime in their
laboratories, whether to research the essence of diseases
or in trying to prevent aging, are mainly concerned with
the chain of events generated by the disintegration of
this membrane. So, what do these scientists study about
this membrane?

*We already said that there is the electron carrier called
cytochrome C on this membrane. If the membrane
disintegrates as a result of free radical damage, cytochrome
C leaks through the mitochondrion. Then the
mitochondrion turns into leaky mitochondrion—which
means there would be holes on the mitochondrion
membrane. This is exactly like the leaky gut.*

Once cytochrome C leaks through mitochondria,
it is too late! *It is the point of no return for the cell.* After
cytochrome C leaks, the cell cannot escape death. *The
cytochrome C leak is the suicide signal of the cell.* This is
what I explained about apoptosis. In this way, we can
see that self-sacrificing apoptosis is controlled by
mitochondria as well.

Self-Sacrificing Mitochondrion

It is the mitochondrion that persuades the damaged cells to destroy themselves voluntarily and enables entropy-resisting, fresh cells to replace them, so that entropy cannot win the battle immediately. What an impressive system, right? Mitochondrion, which works hard to keep the body alive under the most ideal conditions for as long as possible, gets to a point where it sacrifices itself like a kamikaze pilot for the benefit of the whole!

As for the cancerous cell, it assumes it can escape entropy. It does not opt for apoptosis. It says, "why am I to die?!" "What do I care about the benefit of the whole?!" It is selfish. It spreads, it gets stronger; but in the end, it consumes the entire being it resides in, at the expense of its own life!

Healthy cells, on the other hand, sacrifice themselves for the good of the whole.

As I mentioned previously, sometimes apoptosis cannot take place. **We can define a cell that's stuck in the leaky mitochondria state as above that cannot go through apoptosis as chronic inflammation.**

This is the topic behind the research of all those hardworking scientists. So, what happens if the leaking cell cannot destroy itself and remains to leak?

- **chronic diseases**
- **cancer**

In summary, if we overeat and exceed the pace of cycles and flows, if we continuously send nutrients to the cell, there will be:

- an increase in free radicals.
- a decrease in membrane voltage.
- membrane disintegration turning into drug-leaking mitochondria.
- Cytochrome C leakage; self-destruction of the cell.
- a starting point for chronic disease, inflammation, and cancer if the cell cannot commit suicide.

This is how all the diseases you know and don't know of begin...

In summary of the summary above:

- ETC should always flow.
- ATP/ADP cycle should always flow
- NAD/NADH should always flow.
- TCA should always flow.
- If all of the above do not flow or circulate, then it means we're in great trouble.

Eating the Galaxy / The Philosophy of Eating

Before I end this chapter, I want to add something to the topic of why we eat. In fact, when you look at the big picture, do you know why we eat? We eat to capture all that galactic energy! You've probably sensed it by now. In the simplest terms: through consuming plants that photosynthesize and the animals that feed on those plants, we are actually indirectly eating the sunlight.

Photosynthesis is the exact opposite of what we do in the mitochondria. In the plant's ETC, the sunlight's energy separates the electrons and protons of hydrogen found in the water that the plant takes from the soil. Just like us. The chloroplast cell that captures the light is the plant's mitochondria. The chloroplast cell generates proton gradient on its membrane and produces ATP and glucose. Just like us.

While doing this, the plant draws in carbon dioxide and releases oxygen. We do exactly the opposite; photosynthesis and oxidative phosphorylation in human ETC are exactly opposite processes.

Therefore, simply put, we eat in order to obtain the sunlight through plants and animals who eat plants. We acquire our strength from the sun in our resistance against the universe's entropy. For chaos not to win and to preserve order, energy is required. We eat to preserve the order in the organism. Because our real energy source is the sun, we cannot get any energy from processed foods, as they do not possess any sunlight energy!

Although I would like to simplify it as much as possible, my hands are tied due to the complexity of the system. So far, you've learned about the negative effects of overeating. "So, what's next," you may be wondering. I will explain how easily you can gain weight and get haunted by diseases due to malnutrition, even if you do not overeat.

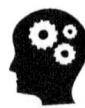

The Cost of an Unhealthy Diet

"A little food, a restful life." —*Turkish Proverb*

In the previous section, we searched for an answer to the question of how much we should eat. There is a cliché response to this question, and you probably have heard it many times. **The amount you should eat is specific to the individual. It depends on the gender, age, level of activity, health issues, and so on.**

These general statements are true. However, since my aim is to explain nutritional biochemistry on a molecular level, I cannot tell you that these are the answers to the questions and put this book aside.

More or less, we now know the answer to how much we are supposed to eat. We all know that we should eat as much as we utilize the ATP we produce. If we cannot utilize ATP, we should not continue to eat. We should eat to preserve the ADP/ATP cycle. We should eat enough so that we prevent electrons from accumulating and being left behind in the ETC.

If we do not do this, then

- the ETC stops,
- the proton pump stops,
- the membrane voltage drops down,
- plenty of free radicals generate,
- the membrane disintegrates,
- a leaky mitochondrion forms,
- the cytochrome C leaks,
- the irreversible signal of death for the cell comes on,
- the cell either dies, or
- the cell makes you sick.

So, if we translate this biochemical data into daily language, the plainest explanation and summary would be this: *eat little and move around!*

In any case, due to the results of hundreds of studies, doctors have come to an agreement on the following: the scientifically proven formula for a longer life is to reduce the amount of daily calorie intake. Therefore, the wisdom in the statement "if you eat less, you live longer" lies in the boring biochemistry lecture I have just delivered in the previous sections.

Moreover, there isn't one doctor that wouldn't stress the value of exercise. You can read about the benefits of exercise for preventing diseases and extending life between the lines of the boring but helpful biochemistry discussions made thus far.

In short, we should eat and exercise enough to allow the continuous flow of the cycles.

Now, let's respond to the question of "how much should we eat?" with regards to topics we are most curious about, such as weight management, obesity, diabetes, and insulin resistance. In this section, again, there are many biochemical references. But, if you've come this far in the book, I assume you have become familiar with them already. In fact, I am certain you'll figure out everything I explain in the blink of an eye (Okay, maybe it's not so easy; but I know you are hardworking readers). Yes, without any further ado, I will return to the topic of weight management.

Gaining Weight: Is It Because You Eat Too Much?

Let's begin with processed flour and sweetened goods we call **simple carbohydrates,** which are forbidden by every doctor and are by far the most blamed items for weight gain. How is it that they are always number one on the perpetrator list? Its name gives it away—simple carbohydrates! What are simple carbohydrates? What are complicated ones, complex carbohydrates, that is?

Here is the explanation: if it's processed and its natural state is altered, if its whole and hard-to-digest state is transformed into half-digested small pieces in a factory, then we call it a simple carbohydrate. For example, what is the original state of flour and sugar?

One comes from grains or legumes, the other from the sugar beet family.

If we consume these plants in their original forms, it would take us much time to digest. A lot of time would need to pass for the food to go from the stomach to the intestines, to the liver, then to be digested and transferred into the blood stream. *This means that the time between you putting the glucose in your mouth and when it reaches the cell will be extended. So, here's our first finding: pace is important! If carbohydrates are not in their natural states—if they're processed, then they mix into the blood stream and knock on the cell's door very quickly.*

Our major concern regarding these carbohydrates is the pace. But, why is it a concern? A few pages ago we discussed that flows and cycles should continue at a certain pace. *Nutrients that arrive faster to the ETC than the electron flow suffocate it as if we've eaten too much even if we've eaten a little.* Electrons in the ETC get clogged, so they cannot flow. If electrons do not flow, protons cannot be kept on the other side of the membrane, and the free radical amount escalates. Gradually, the ETC slows down, and eventually it completely stops. It would be impossible to generate ATP out of the cell's mitochondria.

If we keep eating, the electron carriers NADH and FADH2 that cannot enter the ETC would remain in the TCA and transform into triglycerides, which is fat in the blood. These fats create our weight. While triglycerides are formed, pyruvate that cannot be transported to the mitochondria returns to glycolysis. When glucose burns without oxygen, pyruvate in glycolysis ends up as lactic acid. Lactic acid causes fatigue, and glycolysis barely generates any energy.

Thus, when we consume simple carbohydrates, we clog the ETC and damage the mitochondria. Even if we eat very little, we gain weight and also suffer from energy deprivation. We eat but feel exhausted.

Excess Fuel Waste

Now, you've understood the initial meaning of the recommendation, "do not eat simple carbohydrates." They are transported to the bloodstream very quickly; even if we eat very little, they arrive at the gates of mitochondria very fast. They get charged more quickly than we can consume and clog the flow of the ETC. When free radicals formed as a result of clogging slows down the ETC, these fuels cannot transform into ATP and have no choice but to transform into fat. Consequentially, we gain weight very easily. And, because the energy model forms lactate residue (glycolysis), we feel exhausted. *We eat less, we gain weight, and we feel exhausted.*

Let's remember another detail regarding carbohydrates. Carbohydrates enter the ETC through the first station, Complex 1. *Complex 1 is the station that generates free radicals most frequently.* The ETC slows down immediately here. What I'm saying is that this type of fuel brings out excessive amounts of waste! Processed simple carbohydrates (baked goods, desserts, candy, beverages, instant fructose syrups, etc.) are the active agents in all diseases from diabetes to Alzheimer's, from thyroid disorders to rheumatism, from migraine to cancer, because of this mechanism. They are fuels with excess waste.

Healthy fats enter through Complex 2 and generate less free radicals. Now, let's write down this one critical detail in bold and highlight it with bright colors. If there are simple carbohydrates to enter through Complex 1, no matter how much healthy fat you consume, fats entering through Complex 2 will not transform into energy! They go to the storage. **Why?**

- Because, those that enter through Complex 1 take over the ETC faster. Because, the survival mechanism prefers to burn glucose first, as it is cheap fuel. For instance, olive oil is considered to be a healthy fat. But, if you eat olive oil with simple carbohydrates, instead of with vegetables, glucose is generated instantly and enters through Complex 1. Therefore, instead of being used as energy, olive oil is stored as triglycerides. So, it's not wise to eat simple carbohydrates with olive oil.
- Another important detail is that when you

eat too much simple carbohydrates and disrupt mitochondria membranes with free radicals, you also hinder carnitine in carrying fats through the membranes to be burned in the mitochondria. If carnitine cannot carry fats through the membranes, fats cannot be burned.

In a nutshell, if we want to use fats for energy, then we shouldn't combine them with simple carbohydrates.

Plants give energy while they clear waste with their antioxidants. Since it takes longer to digest complex carbohydrates (grains, nuts, fibrous seeds, and so on, are actually unprocessed plants), they do not knock on ETC's door that fast. But if they are exposed to high temperatures (overcooking, frying, etc.) they reach the ETC faster. Preferably, they should be consumed lightly cooked, or raw and cold.

Ready-made corn syrup usually consists of fructose that easily breaks down. But, fructose in fruit does not break down that easily and delays the fiber entering the bloodstream. Thus, fructose in fruit does not run to knock on the door of the ETC. However, ready-made corn syrup is a problem for it appears at ETC's door in the blink of an eye.

Insulin Resistance: An Issue the World Is Still Unable to Resolve

We need to talk more about obesity and diabetes—both

are results of consuming excessive amounts of simple carbohydrates.

1. I've blamed these nutrients for clogging the ETC's flow because they get into the bloodstream very swiftly.
2. Also, I've pointed out that they enter the ETC through Complex 1, the station that produces the most free radicals.

They disrupt the ETC for the above-mentioned two reasons. The result would be a kind of suffocation, because oxygen is where ETC is utilized. If we cannot use the ETC, then it means we cannot use oxygen either. The hemoglobin A1c test and high values of fasting insulin in diabetes are indications for this hypoxia on a cellular level.

This procedure—identified as the mitochondria's oxygenated breath, as the name suggests, is where breathing takes place. If oxygen is not utilized accurately, then it generates free radicals. As the free radicals increase in number, they harm not only mitochondria but the rest of the cell as well. Free radicals first and foremost damage the membranes. Damage starting at the mitochondria membrane goes further to the outer membrane. If the amount of free radicals is more than the cell's antioxidants are able to clear, then the free radicals have to attack someplace. Free radicals also damage the outer membrane of the cell. The medical term of this is lipid peroxidation, which is the oxidation of the fats inside the membrane. In daily language, we refer to oxidation for rusting; in medical language, it is losing electrons. The opposite, however, is reduction—in other words, the gaining of electrons. The function of free radicals is oxidation, and that of antioxidants is reduction.

In the cells, the oxidation-reduction occurrence has a proportion referred to as the redox balance. If the redox balance is disrupted, membranes are the first to get harmed. After free radicals snatch their electrons, the oxidized cell membranes have a difficult time in communicating with the outer cell, as electron loss causes a kind of deafness. The electric voltage on the membrane gets altered. As with the mitochondria inner membrane, the voltage drops. This shift breaks down the communication between hormones and the cell. Hormones outside communicate with the cell through receptors on this membrane. Insulin is a hormone as well. This is how it works. In an oxidized membrane, its receptors cannot hear the commands of the insulin hormone. The insulin hormone's power over the cell diminishes. The condition known as insulin resistance is something similar to this. The concept insulin resistance is actually an explanation of rusted cell membranes. Furthermore, insulin and the insulin receptor's interaction require a lot of energy. When ATP production in the cell decreases, there isn't sufficient energy. With this sequence of events, everything explained in this book thus far culminates here—at the point of *insulin resistance*!

Insulin resistance is the beginning sign for numerous diseases. In my opinion, what insulin resistance tells us is that there are some errors in energy production, and that a lot of waste is generated during production.

Hence, all metabolic events that use energy are affected by this situation. That's why everywhere we look, insulin resistance appears to be the guilty party. In order not to crave sweets after meals, not to feel hungry constantly, not to gain weight easily, we need to regulate insulin resistance. Do you have any of these complaints? Think carefully.

On the other hand, you should ask yourself, "how is my emotional state?" Observe yourself. If you experience emotional highs and lows before menstruation, anxiety, brain fog, frequent forgetfulness, the solution is to decrease the sugar going to the brain and to break the insulin resistance of brain cells!

If you do not want to have insulin resistance, do the following:

- Produce as much ATP as you can consume.
- Do not eat more than the pace of ADP/ATP cycle.
- Do not consume foods that would clog the ETC flow.

If you don't follow this advice, everything you eat will

be stored as triglycerides—which is fat, and your cell membranes will be oxidized and go deaf. Because your insulin will increase, you will constantly be hungry and eat.

This last sentence is probably a familiar one for many of you. Insulin resistance is not just an issue of diabetes; it is the sign that the cell's energy metabolism is beginning to malfunction. Our choice of food and eating at times that are inappropriate for our circadian rhythm increase insulin resistance rapidly. Now, we often see that children and teenagers also suffer from insulin resistance. There is almost no one unaffected by insulin resistance. Insulin resistance is perhaps the greatest "gift" to us by modern life. I'm sure you know that I used the word "gift" ironically! The major source of free radicals, which generate lipid oxidization on the cell membrane and are the molecular cause of insulin resistance, is the mitochondria in the body. And processed food is the trigger. But, modern life gives us free radicals not only through food but by other means as well. Environmental toxins, stress, certain types of lifestyle cause us to become oxidized. Thus, we are damaged by free radicals from the outside as well as from the inside.

Nevertheless, let's remember the errors of the energy metabolism every time we hear the term "free radicals." Insulin resistance—the initial determinant—can be seen in polycystic ovary syndrome as well. Metabolic syndrome also has insulin resistance. There might be insulin resistance in heart diseases. It's seen in fatty liver disease. Obesity and diabetes have insulin resistance. In Alzheimer's, insulin resistance can also be detected. In fact, many chronic diseases advance hand in hand with insulin resistance.

It seems that insulin resistance is the first stage of the cellular degeneration that can be measured in the lab. *If there is insulin resistance, it means that in the mitochondrion of that specific cell, things aren't going well.*

Treatment Options For Insulin Resistance

For many years now, the first treatment option for insulin resistance has been drugs containing metformin. If you're curious about how they work and want to read about it, you might come across the following expressions in medical statements:

- It decreases the amount of electrons entering Complex 1 (it would be as if you ate very little).
- It works by a system that has the letters AMP in it.

What is AMP?

AMP is adenosine mono-one-phosphate. It's ATP with one phosphate.

When, as a result of malnutrition, the ETC gets clogged and ADPs cannot transform into ATP and therefore accumulate, then the body brings together two ADPs for emergency energy situations. It generates a three-phosphate ATP and leaves behind that one phosphate AMP, which is adenosine monophosphate.

ADP+ADP=ATP+AMP

In this way, ADPs decrease and become ATP, but AMPs increase.

In other words, in malfunctions of advanced levels of energy production, AMP escalates. **The existence of AMP is the alarm that indicates an energy deficiency in the cell.** It is a signal that increases the body's craving for food. That's why the drug used for diabetes and insulin resistance is metformin; it affects AMP.

Having excessive amounts of AMP lying around triggers a path to aging called *mTOR*. You shouldn't be surprised when you hear statements from the medical community such as "the inventor of the drug preventing mTOR will succeed in extending the human lifespan." There are insane numbers of research studies taking place on blocking mTOR activity in cancer mechanisms. It seems as though AMP and mTOR paths are troublemakers in a fundamental way.

This path, the mTOR path, is a signal that belongs to the regressing cell. When the mitochondrion is damaged, it is the DNA in the nucleus that sees the AMPs escalating. As a solution, it gives a command to go into a metabolic shift. To increase the reduced energy levels caused by the AMPs, which indicate the malfunctioning of the mitochondrion, oxygen-free energy production through glycolysis is initiated in order to save the cell. This signal, the mTOR signal, is the signal that the cell goes into energy production by fermentation, resulting in lactic acid. Since we are complicated beings, this method does not provide us with enough energy for long. It's a short-term solution. One of the effects of metformin is to decrease the AMP path and the mTOR signal.

What metformin really does is to lower the amount of carbohydrates entering through Complex 1. But, if you read its side effects, very little increase in lactic acid could be mentioned. Readers who are savvy in reading the prospectus will remember this immediately. Because when electrons cannot enter Complex 1, metformin also seems to trigger the lactate path.

However, if you think you can continue to eat simple carbohydrates as you always have and resolve matters with the help of metformin, it's not a hundred-percent-guaranteed solution. The effects of metformin have been the subject of innumerable PubMed studies for almost thirty years now. And, metformin is still the first choice for insulin resistance. It's use is common and safe.

To make things simpler, let me explain nutrition through a fuel and combustion analogy. The fuel you put in your car's engine (mitochondrion) clogs the pipes (ETC). The engine is not working to its fullest level (oxygen cannot be used) and burns fuel by emitting smoke (free radicals and lactate). This might not be a problem for two kilometers, but when you go further down the road, the cell fills up with enough free radicals to kill itself. The car needs a new engine. If we insist on running the car and feeding it with poor fuel, then even the hood of the car starts to decay (hood=cell membrane). Now, imagine a brand new, shiny car; and next to it an old, worn out, rusty car. That's how the new and old cells look. In order to remain shiny and brand new, we've already learned how much we should eat and what we should eat.

We have now returned to the critical question I have already partially answered and is the actual reason this book was written.

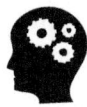

Chapter 3:

"When you eat, look at your watch not at your plate."—
Dr. A. Ç.

I have explained in detail since the beginning of this book, that we have to eat according to the circadian rhythm. I emphasized that circadian hormones affect our bodies in various ways during the day and at night. Now, let's have a look at how our energy centers—the mitochondria—function in line with the circadian clock. Just to make things more intriguing, it might be a good idea to mention the two circadian rhythms of the mitochondria, which were discovered in 2004:

- Coenzyme Q10 is at its highest at 3:27 p.m., and at its lowest at 10:00 p.m.. What is Coenzyme Q10? It's a carrier that carries electrons from carbohydrates in Complex 1 and electrons from fats in Complex 2 to Complex 3 in the electron transport chain, forms ATP, and burns what we eat.

- The electron transport chain's first station Complex 1, which also burns carbohydrates, functions at its peak from 09:02 in the morning until 2:22 in the afternoon. Its functions slow down as of 4:21 in the afternoon.

If we put these two statements next to each other, we could more or less get the picture: *We understand when we can burn food and transform it into ATP, and when we cannot generate ATP and gain weight. Right?*

Of course, the only price we pay for overeating and eating at the wrong time does not merely consist of gaining weight. It is also the increase in free radicals and leaky mitochondria as a result of the disruption in the electron transport chain. I tried to explain all of this in the previous chapters. If ATP is not used, the production stops, and the AMP/ADP/ATP proportions are disturbed.

Between ATP production and the ETC, there are basically three alternatives:

- If you eat little, there will be less electrons entering the ETC; then the ETC does not get clogged, and there are no free radicals.

114

- If you eat a lot but exercise, ATP that is produced gets used; again, the ETC does not get clogged, and there are no free radicals.
- If you eat a lot and do not exercise, then free radicals will take over.

Now, it's time to add the missing link, the circadian rhythm, to all this data we have. If you eat at night, even if you eat very little, it is a problem. Because at night, our biological clock is set for nutrient starvation. When we look at the times Complex 1 is actively functioning, we see the significance of the question "when should we eat?" Complex 1 is the first station carbohydrates enter the ETC; but the main feature of Complex 1 is that it produces the most free radicals.

Complex 1 begins to get incompetent around 5:00 p.m., actually, somewhere as of 4:20 p.m. and onwards. Especially after 5:00 p.m., if we overeat, we will obviously cause it to produce free radicals instead of ATP. *We know that particularly simple carbohydrates, which are relentlessly knocking on the mitochondria door, will cause free radical damage, even if they don't create weight problems. This is all due to the circadian settings.*

Even if we do not gain weight, and even if it doesn't do much harm in the short-term, we trigger a chain reaction that would come back and haunt us as a variety of illnesses. In the evening, since mitochondria do not want to function and burn carbohydrates, they slow down Complex 1. This is again for survival. The energy-producing system is not for functioning during the night.

At night, mitochondria leaks decrease. If ETC food intake is reduced during the night, then the number of free radicals is reduced, as well. Mitochondria become reductive, and this means they will be charged with negative voltage. Reduction is the opposite of oxidation. In case of oxidation, negative charge decreases, and positive charge increases. In case of reduction, negative charge increases, and positive charge decreases.

Throughout the night, as the amount of free radicals is reduced, and because mitochondria membrane has more negative voltage, the electric charge will increase. This is a good voltage that reduces leaky mitochondria. But during the day, the free radicals cause this voltage to diminish, since free radicals harm the mitochondria membrane and increase the possibility of membrane leaks. Therefore, there's more mito leak during the day with a reduction at night. We know that the more leaks there are in the mitochondria, the faster we age.

Since mitochondrial leaks can go from the leaky gut to blood-brain barrier leaks, all sorts of leaks subside at night. All barriers and borders are repaired. But of course, only if we do not eat and sleep on time. *At night, Complex 1, which is the path of carbohydrates, is shut down. But still, energy is needed for metabolism to function. For obtaining that energy, our fats in the storage are used. Here is the formula to losing weight while we sleep.*

How Do We Burn Fat While We Sleep?

There are two ways that ETC obtains electrons from food:

1. Electrons that come from carbohydrates via NADH
2. Electrons that come from fats via FADH2

NADH enters the ETC through Complex 1; FADH2, through Complex 2. *The purpose of Complex 1 slowing down at night is to allow fat electrons to come from Complex 2 via FADH2.*

This is important for 2 reasons:

1. No free radicals are produced in Complex 2. This is good for cells that will be clearing the body of free radicals with antioxidants throughout the night.
2. The fats we would like to receive via FADH2 are the fats the body stored, not the fats received from food. During nighttime starvation, the body wants to get rid of the unwanted fats around the internal organs and blood fats, such as

> high levels of triglycerides in the blood,
> by transforming them into energy.

Internal organ lipoidosis is a common condition that operates like a type of endocrine disease; it can be detected by the naked eye in the increase of waist-hip proportions. These fats release substances that cause inflammation.

Studies show that by eating less, longevity cells SIRT are activated. Eating at night deactivates SIRT cells. This means that if you eat at night, you can forget about having a long life. But, in my opinion, another aspect that activates these longevity cells is the work of Complex 2. Complex 2, other than being the complex that burns fats, also has another characteristic: although it is Mito-DNA that manages all ETC complexes, Complex 2 is managed by the nucleus DNA.

What do I mean by this?

I've explained that mitochondria have their own DNAs and that they are rather plenty in number. So much so that the DNA numbers of mitochondria are ten to twenty times higher than our nucleus DNA.

Why are they so many? They are for the following reason: mitochondria want to make their own decisions as fast as possible. MitoDNA carries the required genes that belong to Complexes 1, 3, 4, and 5. Their management has nothing to do with our nucleus DNA. However, Complex 2 is managed by the main DNA. Also, longevity genes are in the main DNA. From my point of view, Complex 2–where the body fats get burned and is a signal for nutrient starvation—activates the SIRT genes, which are the longevity genes in our DNA.

This theory of mine makes sense. If we think about the times of famine, when there is not enough food, bodily fats get burned. This is a signal for starvation. The body has preserved its survival sense for thousands of years by activating genes that would protect its life. The DNA, which already works in a circadian manner, knows that as it gets dark in the evening, the living creature will wait hungry in a corner for the day to rise, while burning their own bodily fats throughout the night.

As the night falls, burning unnecessary fats is clean fuel (glucose is dirty fuel) for the metabolism that repairs itself during the night; it also provides what is required for a long life by activating SIRT genes. As it burns the unwanted fats around the organs, it also uses damaged, unwanted cells as spare parts during this process. It provides fuel for good and vital cells as well as missing parts from old cells. It works as a sort of a recycling system; in other words, it performs autophagy.

In the next chapter, we will look for answers to the question, "how do we eat?" When I say "how," I mean the process prior to reaching the cell; the journey of the bite that starts in the mouth.

Chapter 4:

"On a long and narrow road, I walk."—Aşık Veysel

In this chapter, we will examine the journey of food starting from the mouth until it knocks on the cell's door—like a film, scene by scene. Perhaps, in other books, you've read about this journey already. But, the difference here is that beyond sharing with you the known facts, I aim to connect these facts with mitochondria, cell health, and the internal circadian clock.

From the moment you put a morsel in your mouth to the moment it reaches the cell, there are things you can do to obtain clean energy; but, after it gets to the cell, the situation is out of your hand. Therefore, I would like to remind you that I will be discussing food choices in the next chapter and would like to reserve this chapter to the details of how we can support the digestive system. As I said, perhaps you have heard much information on this topic; however, the way it's explained here will lead to some different perceptions. Trust me.

I sometimes think about this thing called digestion, and what long and demanding work it has. Couldn't we have a much shorter way of obtaining energy from food? The answer is hidden in biochemistry once again. Digestion is not only about the end result, which is the intake of food; it is a perfectly planned system that provides benefits at every stage.

Let's start with the mouth. Naturally, we cannot begin to talk about it without emphasizing the **importance of chewing**. Chewing breaks down nutrients chemically through the enzymes inside the mouth, and mechanically through the teeth. **Saliva secretion in the mouth is circadian**. While there is more saliva secretion during the day, at night it decreases. That's the reason why we wake up with our mouth dry in the morning.

There is absorption through the mouth as well. The inner mucosa of the mouth, which seems not to have any other tasks to undertake, actually absorbs some of the nutrients, immediately. For instance, there are many sublingual pills that we use. The sublingual area is where there is direct entrance, and where matter gets quickly absorbed. When we chew food, many of the substances inside are transported to the blood through this place. If we especially chew on plants and fresh food longer, vitamins and minerals as well as good fats will be transported into the bloodstream through the sublingual region. Personally, when I eat vegetables and fruits, I try to keep them in my mouth for long periods of time. I do the same for fats as well. Therefore, they are easily transported to the bloodstream. I also do it to protect the mucosa of the mouth.

Inside the mouth, there is also a barrier, a borderline. Our intestines are known to be the border between us and nutrients. However, we do not consider that the same relates to the mouth. Actually, it is sensible to consider the zone between our mouth and anus as external rather than internal. A pipe goes through us, and that is our surface of contact to the outside world. Lungs, the nose, and skin are also our surface of contact. These are our borders. *In the end, all stomach-intestine issues, with which we are familiar regarding cases about nutrition, are the result of the invasion of these borders by false nutrients or false bacteria.*

The invasion expression just fits perfectly, here! I suppose there isn't one single person that has not experienced the invasion of borders, who has not experienced the troubles created by invaders, despite all the power we possess concerning the protection of our borders. Even if we procure all the best health conditions, even if we have no complaints, the borders mentioned above can be disrupted by an external impact, by an allergy, by antibiotics, by a tooth cavity, or by stress. Throughout our lives, one of our major concerns should be to preserve these borders. However, these borders are not made of steel; they are made of cells. In order for cells to protect the borders, to keep mucosa sturdy, to provide digestion and absorption, and to maintain all these processes, they need mitochondria that can produce outstanding energy.

For maintaining strength of mucosa cells in the mouth, I would like to emphasize the *importance of consuming fibrous plants and fats.* As you chew on plants and make contact with fats such as coconut oil, these cells preserve their strength. Gums of our teeth are also mucosa. It shouldn't be too difficult to figure out that if our teeth and gum health are not good, then bacteria can easily enter through. Bleeding of the gum indicates that there is trouble with mucosa, and the mouth-bacteria border is not strong. We generally tend to neglect the fact that our teeth and gum health are the beginning points of our holistic health. For example, *there may be infectious foci in the roots of teeth due to a root canal procedure. There are publications that consider these infections as an increasing risk factor for heart diseases and diseases such as breast cancer.* These are again easy areas for invaders trying to push their way in to violate our borders. Of course, these are topics of dentists; but, I only would like to highlight the establishment of border protection, designating the external and internal areas in our mouths.

LPS, which we will mention while we're discussing the intestines, are also transported to the bloodstream through the mouth. You may not know about these LPS just yet; however, I assume you will be shocked when you read the chapter where I will be discussing the ways in which they can cause us trouble. Now, leaving general oral health to dentists, let's go back to cellular health.

Chewing on fibrous plants long and consuming fats such as butter and coconut oil protect the mucosa of the mouth and regenerate it, as they do with the mucosa cells of the intestines. Inside the mouth is an oxygenated environment. The presence of anaerobic bacteria of tooth abscesses inside the mouth is not welcome. However, inside the intestines is an oxygen-free environment. *I wonder whether we disrupt the oxygen-free environment of the intestines when we eat and swallow too fast?* Would eating fast and swallowing air decrease the number of bacteria in the intestines? Food for thought. Yet, we should eat slowly anyway for a relaxed digestion.

Eating slowly decreases the amount of energy that is digested and transported into the bloodstream per unit of time. For someone who eats the same amount of food more quickly, glucose will reach the cell more quickly as well. Remember, we don't want more glucose than we can consume knocking at the door of the ETC during energy production, as this increases the number of free radicals and causes fats to be stored. *Therefore, eating slowly activates a similar system as nutrient starvation in the body.* When we eat slowly, weight-gaining signals do not function. Since this slow pace of food intake will not clog the flow of the electron transport chain, the ideal pace of NAD/NADH and AMP/ADP/ATP will be preserved.

This is the same as preserving mitochondria. The chain of events that cause leaky mitochondria in consequence of a clogged ETC will not be triggered.

Whatever the disease in question might be, eating slowly will support the healing process of that condition, because the mitochondria are protected. *Even if you are not to follow any of the nutritional advice, you will at least benefit from increasing the number of times you chew your food.* When you're too ill to eat anything, your doctor will ask you to count your morsels. Instead of your doctor asking you to count your morsels, you should begin counting the number of times you chew your food, so you won't need a doctor.

One of the functions of the stomach is to digest protein. Animal or plant-based, the digestion of protein takes place here. Digesting protein is more difficult than digesting carbohydrates. The PH of stomach acid is the most acidic in the body, and it is important to preserve this value in order to digest protein. *Most people have a lack of stomach acid. It requires a whole lot of energy to pump the necessary amount of acid into the stomach from the stomach wall.* You should be familiar with the preventatives of acid known as proton pump inhibitors. These protons are the foundations of stomach acid. Outstanding stomach cell mitochondria are required in order for these to be pumped into the stomach from the stomach wall.

If a person is unaware that they're lacking stomach acid, they will have difficulty in digesting the protein consumed, especially in the evenings. When undigested protein gets to the intestines, and if there is leaky gut syndrome as well, then the protein may infiltrate inside. These undigested proteins are considered foreign bodies by the immune system and are one of the main issues regarding our problems with food. Especially, the lack of digestion of proteins such as meat, milk, and cheese can cause unwanted sensitivity in the body.

We should give some external support, chew well what we eat, and not consume heavy proteins in the evenings if stomach acidity is insufficient. If acid in the stomach is less than what is required, then plant-based nutrients may cause problems as well. Generally, harmless bacteria that come with vegetables and fruits die in stomach acid. However, if stomach acidity is insufficient, then the remaining bacteria may be transmitted to the small intestines and cause problems with bloating and gas. *To prevent this condition—also known as sibo, to decrease the bacteria population in the upper parts of the intestine, and to support stomach acid, it is recommended that we consume large amounts of lemon and apple cider vinegar at meals and wash vegetables well.*

Reflux—another digestive problem—can be defined as the laxity of the pharynx lower lid. When you swallow, you swallow air as well. Swallowing air is not desirable for the oxygen-free environment of the intestine. Eating slowly might be a solution, however.

Insufficient stomach acid is also a problem for the

absorption of vitamin B12 and iron. This should be considered in cases of anemia. The duodenum, which is located under the stomach, does not have a protective shield for acid as the stomach does. When nutrients that are mixed with stomach acid arrive at the duodenum— in other words, the small intestines, high levels of stomach acid are neutralized here by the carbonate-consisting pancreatic fluid. The more we consume animal products, the more the stomach will try to produce acid. Moreover, in order to neutralize the acid after passing through the stomach, the pancreas will produce that much pancreatic alkaline fluid.

In addition to the alkaline fluid, the pancreas produces enzymes to digest the incoming nutrients. There are enzymes to digest fats, carbohydrates, and proteins. You may take digestive enzyme supplements under the supervision of a doctor to balance the pancreatic enzyme deficiency. Furthermore, we know that the pancreas releases insulin. In fact, the beta cells of the pancreas secrete insulin. **Beta cells are circadian.** They want to function according to the rhythms of day and night. Increasing blood sugar levels by eating at night and forcing the pancreas to secrete insulin at the wrong time is inappropriate.

It is important to know that there are a limited number of mitochondria in **pancreatic** beta cells. If the amount of mitochondria in these cells is low, then it means that their capacity to produce high levels of energy is low as well. Thus, where does that lead us? If they can't find high levels of energy, then they get tired easily while functioning. Eating in the evening exhausts the pancreatic beta cells. Nutrients and the ways of eating mentioned in the paragraphs above disrupt the pancreas. On the other hand, a plant-based diet does not exhaust the pancreas.

The gallbladder only gets your attention in sentences such as "I have gallstones/gallbladder sludge," but, the gallbladder is a very valuable organ. First of all, it's one of the detoxing organs. Toxins that occur in the liver and need to be eliminated by feces arrive at the intestines through the gallbladder. The objective of the fluid known as gallbladder fluid is to absorb the fat that comes into the intestines via nutrients. It is important for the gallbladder to open up and gallbladder fluid to pour into the gut for the absorption of fats and the absorption of vitamins that dissolve in fats. While this takes place, toxin wastes coming from the liver are sent to the intestines.

The neck of the gallbladder should be lax, not contracted. On the contrary to common knowledge, laxity requires more energy than contraction. So, if the mitochondria's ATP production is low, the gallbladder cells will find it difficult to gather the energy to loosen up. For the gallbladder neck to unwind, we need "ATP money." Otherwise, toxins that the gallbladder cannot expel will return to the liver and line up to be cleaned again—thus, increasing the amount of work undertaken by the liver. If we are talking about liver detoxification, we should remember that one of the ways to eliminate toxins is through the gallbladder. We often hear that the intestines, the kidneys, the skin, the lungs, and the liver are toxin-eliminating organs, while the gallbladder is treated like a stepchild. The more we eat fibrous foods and good fats, the more relaxed the gallbladder neck becomes. Chili is also a good choice in making the gallbladder neck function and extract enzymes.

Let's come to **the liver**. Everything we put in our mouths stops by this metabolizing factory, where toxins go through two stages of detoxification. You may find the details in my previous books. For now, we can review some simple eating recommendations, in order to benefit more from the phase 1 and phase 2 of the stages of detoxification. Here are some of these recommendations: nutrients of broccoli, cauliflower, and cabbage groups; turmeric; ginger; berberine type of spices; all B vitamins; fresh fruits and vegetables containing vitamin C; dark purple fruits and vegetables containing anthocyanin; foods that boost glutathione such as artichoke and thistle; foods containing cysteine such as onion, garlic, whey; and foods containing selenium. These nutrients support the liver's detoxification process. These plant-based nutrients, which we should always consume more than processed food and not only when we are ill, are very beneficial for the liver. All in all, most plants support the detoxification phases of the liver.

During detoxification of toxic substances, drugs, pesticides, processed foods, preservatives, even the lipstick particles we swallow, our liver is actually in need of extra electrons for cleaning. *Basically, detoxification is carried out by electrons.* (The NADPH molecule in plants—not NADH—is a fundamental reducing agent; in other words, an electron donor. Electron donors and antioxidants are one and the same.)

In the liver, systems that carry out the basic detoxifying procedures operate inside the mitochondria. That's why the cleaner the fuel the liver mitochondria uses, the higher the performance of the detoxification will be. We should remember that the fatty liver condition is caused by consuming too much processed floury and sugary foods, and really grasp that feeding on these types of food for long periods of time damages the liver cells—first the mitochondria and then the entire cell. Processed carbohydrates cause leaky mitochondria in the liver and decrease the production of energy. But, the decrease of mitochondria functioning in the liver means the decrease of the liver's detoxing function. We already know that we need to avoid toxins in order to protect the liver. The first thing that comes to mind as toxins are chemicals and heavy metals. Substances in drugs, painkillers, antibiotics, and various synthetic molecules have a toxic affect on the liver mitochondria. Looking at the list of toxins, it's impossible not to panic for our liver, which carries out the entire cleansing process.

However, we should remember that processed floury and sugary foods are at the top of the liver's toxins list. The liver functions both according to the circadian rhythm and the time that the food enters the body. The liver does not prefer to produce energy and detoxify at the same time. The night and nutrient starvation are more suitable for detoxification.

Although the upper limit for a GGT test, which is required to check the liver functions, is indicated as 60, we should approach it in a "lower the better" kind of manner. *The GGT shows how well the liver uses glutathione reserves of the body in order to cleanse the toxins. Glutathione is the master antioxidant.* GGT levels increase especially through alcohol consumption, as alcohol is a toxin for the liver.

On the other hand, we now know that those who do not consume alcohol suffer non-alcoholic fatty liver as a result of consuming too much simple carbohydrates. We also understand that the liver mitochondria get damaged because of these foods and thus become leaky mitochondria.

Speaking of leaky mitochondria, let's take a look at the leaky gut as well.

Leaky Gut

We know that the intestine wall structure is folded in order to expand the surface area, and that it's called villus. This villus with its indented structure expands the surface, which functions as a barrier between the outside—where there is food and bacteria—and the inside of the body. Remember that the inner membrane of the mitochondria has a similar folded structure as well. The goal is, again, the same. Let's put more surface area in a small place, so that we have an extended area to do more work!

Cells that form the villus of intestines are tightly attached to one another in order to not allow uncontrolled access. It is also called *tight junction*. When the intestines are damaged, this tight junction loosens, and substances that should not go in get access inside. This is what is called the leaky gut. The zonulin test determines whether there is a leak or not. Furthermore, what we see as leaky gut when looking from afar is actually leaky mitochondria if we get closer. Just as all roads lead to Rome, in sickness and in health, all roads lead to the mitochondria!

The inner surface of the intestines is formed of single layered cells. Can you imagine single cells, tightly attached to each other, struggling to protect the whole area? They also decide who gets to have access. The entire security barrier consists of this line of slender, single layer of cells.

Allowing in wanted substances and trying to remain sturdy in order to prohibit unwanted substances from penetrating costs a whole lot of energy for these cells. These cells are no different than the others. They work via ATP as well. After all, this thing called ATP is not produced in one part of the body and sent to wherever it's required! Every cell produces their own ATP, locally. There is no such thing as an ATP importation taking place. Therefore, these cells produce their own ATP to execute all their functions and keep themselves intact.

Let's remember how the cell produces ATP:

- through glycolysis and
- inside the mitochondria.

Yet still, the source of ATP for these cells is the food we eat. Hence, the healthy and unhealthy choices of food directly affect the functions of these barrier cells. If we mainly eat simple carbohydrates and processed foods, this cheap fuel will increase the free radical damage. As a result of leaky mitochondria damaged by free radicals, the ATP production of these cells will come to a stop. Cells that do not function will be eliminated by apoptosis or mitophagy, and new ones will take their place.

The production/destruction cycle of the intestinal wall cells is very fast. These cells are not durable and are entirely renewed every four to five days. The ones that get old are replaced with new ones. We've observed that malnutrition causes this cycle to be generated more quickly. If malnutrition continues, cells that cannot be renewed will keep operating with their damaged mitochondria. Once the cells that are exclusive of apoptosis remain chronically damaged, inflammation on the intestinal wall will appear. As the name indicates, all intestinal disorders are called chronic inflammatory intestinal diseases. Since the way you eat does not change, constant free radical damage takes place. This is what makes it chronic. There are wounds, cracks, and holes on a micro level that cannot heal. This is what makes it inflammatory. *Leaky gut consists of cells full of leaky mitochondria.*

Most hormones produced in the intestines are circadian, and there are different hormones that function during the day and at night. You must've heard many times about the roles of these hormones between the brain and the intestines. *The circadian growth hormone, when released at night, enables intestinal cells to be renewed during sleep.* Sleep deprivation, however, decreases cell renewal. As a result, leaky gut complaints increase; cracks open on the intestinal mucosa.

Now, let's talk about LPS, which would create problems not only in the intestines but everywhere in the body, even in the brain if leaks go through these cracks.

LPS/Our New Health Issue

LPS is defined as lipopolysaccharides. They are a type of fatty structure. This fatty structure is *the structure of gram-negative bacteria membranes.* They are also referred as endotoxins. Therefore, when we refer to LPS, we refer to the waste of dead gram-negative bacteria's outer membrane, which are perceived as toxins wandering around.

Gram-negative bacteria membranes are similar to mitochondria membranes. Bacteria produce ATP on this membrane as well. And yes, bacteria also have ETC on this membrane; they also produce their ATP to stay alive, just like us. Since a bacterium's outer membrane is not folded like that of the mitochondrion inner membrane, they are living creatures producing little amount of energy on a narrow surface. Hence, they have a short lifespan.

When these bacteria die, endotoxins—in other words, LPS—can easily penetrate through the gaps caused by a leaky gut. LPS leaking in are considered as an attack by the immune system cells wherever they are. Endo-toxins is the name. Do I need to say more? They are utterly antigenic for the immune system; there is a "shoot on sight" command for LPS, as the immune system wants to destroy them. As dead bacteria, LPS leaks in through the intestines and can reach any part of the body. They stimulate our immunity everywhere. *They cause chronic inflammation on a micro level and intensify the effects of all inflammatory diseases.*

They can climb up to the brain not only via blood, but also through the vagus nerve that exists between the brain and the intestines. The vagus nerve is the part of the digestive system that goes directly to the brain. It is the communication line between the brain and the intestines. LPS that climb up the vagus nerve reach the blood-brain barrier. We are talking about another barrier, yet again. The barrier between the blood and the brain is extremely tight. It is one of the most solid barriers. After all, the brain is the main command center, and it should be protected! However, considering there are also cells that experience events I've been discussing throughout the entire book, if the mitochondria there gets damaged, then we can talk about leaky mitochondria in that area as well—which would be leaky brain.

Ultimately, LPS coming from the vagus and entering through the leaking barrier cause inflammation inside the brain as well. The inflammatory response is the war and the battlefield is where the attack takes place as a result of a "shoot-on-sight" command.

Chronic diseases are related to the penetration of LPS. As leaky gut advances, the amount of LPS increases, and, in parallel, inflammatory and autoimmune diseases develop. In my opinion, because of the fact that LPS originate from the gram-negative bacteria membrane and have similarities with the mitochondria originating from two-million-year-old bacteria, it can be confusing for the immune system. In the plan of attack the immune system prepares for LPS, the two-layered mitochondria can be confused for the cell's outer membrane, and thus it can miss the target. What gives me this idea is that the intensity of autoimmune diseases, which is the immune system attacking itself, decreases as the health of the intestine is protected.

To protect the intestine barrier cells in order not to give passage to LPS is about protecting their mitochondria. If the mitochondria are preserved and do not leak, then no other leakage will occur. *Putting aside LPS, which are the wastes of intestinal bacteria, friendly bacteria known as probiotics also work according to the circadian rhythm.* Different types of bacteria increase at night and during the day. If we deviate from our rhythm, they will too. The constipation from which we suffer while traveling might be due to the rhythm of friendly bacteria becoming disrupted.

In this chapter, I wanted to remind you that protecting the intestinal mitochondria equals to protecting the health of the intestine. I would like to add the following suggestions on the protection of the intestines:

1. Consume less simple carbohydrates and heavy proteins.
2. Do not eat in the evenings.
3. Eat slowly and chew several times.
4. Consume fibrous nutrients.

The Importance of Fibrous Food in Preventing Leaky Gut Mitochondria

To tell you the truth, the emphasis put on probiotics should actually be transferred to fibrous foods. Why? *The reason is if there is fiber, then bacteria will produce butyric acid from it.* Butyric acid is a type of butter. Even when we eat vegetables, we can generate butter from fiber. This butter is both an energy source for beneficial bacteria and also an energy source for the closest intestinal wall cells.

If a cell uses Complex 1, which is the station carbohydrates enter, it will produce excessive amounts of free radicals. But, if it uses Complex 2–the station that fats enter, then it will produce much less free radicals. With this knowledge, we can understand that the butyric acid produced by beneficial bacteria is the best possible fuel for the intestinal wall cells. Because it is fat, it produces higher levels of energy compared to glucose; and, intestinal wall cells need a lot of ATP while giving access to food and vitamins.

Nutrients cannot be absorbed all at once; they need to be carried inside. The carrying part, called active transport, requires a whole lot of ATP energy. These ATPs are not gathered from afar; they should be produced within the cell that will do the work. You may hear discussions relating to insufficient nutrients, vitamins, or iron from time to time. With regards, several solutions are usually offered. If the ATP production is insufficient in the cells over the surfaces that would absorb nutrients, then there may not be enough energy for these transports to carry inside the food and vitamins. Increasing energy in the intestinal mitochondria makes the transport of insufficient vitamins easier. This is another way to look at it.

Fiber is the most crucial substance for the intestinal

barrier. If there is fiber, then bacteria will gradually multiply and produce butyrate. This fat will then transform into high, waste-free fuel inside the intestinal cells' mitochondria, protect the intestinal wall, prevent LPS penetration, and provide enough energy to carry out the active transport required to absorb nutrients and vitamins. *To summarize, if mitochondria do not leak, then the gut will not leak either.*

We should particularly have a look into which foods damage this area. I have been repeating that floury foods with gluten have a negative affect on our health since my book *We are Full but Starving (Tokuz Ama Açız)* was published in 2012. Gluten protein is an added protein that helps floury goods such as bread to rise. In short, the initial problem it creates is the following: gluten becomes very difficult to digest.

The second issue is that it has high antigenic aspects. It might create a local inflammation on the intestinal wall with the immune reaction it creates. Marker immunity cells, which are types of immunity cells, attach to each other through gluten. We identify these as immune complexes. They should be destroyed. Otherwise, other cells of the immune system will be on the attack. Therefore, the agent is marked, then targeted, and finally destroyed.

Marked immune complexes do not stay within the intestines; they can move around the body. Since wherever they go they are attacked in order to be destroyed, they may also cause damage in the organ at which they arrive. With this short explanation, I'm ending the topic on gluten. But for now, we are able to visualize the connection between chronic diseases and gluten.

If we go back to the intestinal barrier, the destruction operation I mentioned above will, naturally, first take place here. This situation makes it difficult for intestinal walls to remain intact. The first line of defense consisting of one-layered cells can easily get damaged.

The fundamental issue is nutrients containing gluten are simple carbohydrates that are digested very quickly and get to the ETC very quickly. These two groups are generally the same nutrients. You probably remember what I mean by simple carbohydrates or complex carbohydrates. Simple carbohydrates are transported to the bloodstream easily, while complex carbohydrates take a longer time to be transported to the blood, as digesting them takes longer. If you connect these to the cycles of energy production, you will also remember that simple carbohydrates overwhelm the cycle.

Yet, do not be over-delighted once you hear the statement claiming that complex carbohydrates are good. Do not dream of pastries and cakes! We are not talking about floury foods. When we say complex carbohydrates, we mean food containing fiber: legumes, nuts, fruits, vegetables, and so on. These foods' fibrous content is transformed into fat by intestinal bacteria. Eating a plant-based diet, even for just a few weeks, would allow the new intestinal cells to produce better energy by using this fat.

Probiotics Generate Electricity

I want to add to this section an important detail that you have probably not come across before. First, we already know that beneficial bacteria aid our digestion because they ferment nutrients. In a manner of speaking, they make pickles out of them. *But, the fermentation process is actually an electricity-generating process.* Bacteria generating electricity is a newly discovered topic. This electricity is sort of a biophoton. It speaks for itself: bio=alive; photon=light; and light means electricity. Light and electricity can be transformed into each other.

Bacteria generating electricity is similar to our breathing of oxygen. We breathe oxygen in order to take possession of the nutritive electrons present in the air. Since there is no oxygen in the intestines, bacteria need something else to hold on to that are electrons. This is generally iron.

There are studies that associate chronic iron deficiency with an unwanted bacteria population in the intestines. Bacteria's electron flow takes place on the bacteria membrane. The electron flow on gram-positive bacteria's one-layered outer membrane can be determined from outside as an electric signal. This simple ETC chain on the bacteria membrane is where electrons and biophotons are generated. In any case, it is mostly gram-positive bacteria that provide fermentation. This bacterial production of electricity can be widely seen in pickle, yogurt, and kefir production.

Here are some questions we should be considering:

- Could fermented foods be recommended because bacteria generate electricity during the process of fermentation?
- Could fibrous foods be recommended because bacteria produce butyric acid—which is SCFA fat—out of these?
- Could gluten-free foods be recommended to reduce the effects of the damage on immune complexes, local or afar?
- Could floury, sweet, or processed simple carbohydrates not be recommended in order not to overwhelm the ETC of intestinal cells?

When the ETC is overwhelmed, the generation of energy is taken over by lactic acid. If this happens often, leaky gut advances. When it becomes more chronic, IBS develops. IBS is sometimes associated with diarrhea and mostly with constipation.

The reason constipation is common on a cellular level is the insufficient mitochondrial ATP of intestinal muscle cells. Intestinal muscles are muscles that we call smooth muscles, and are not consciously controlled like the arm muscles. Moreover, they are under the control of the parasympathetic system, functioning involuntarily. The intestine's contraction and release are controlled by this system. Constipation can be defined as intestinal muscles remaining contracted. Normal defecation requires for the intestinal muscles to have regular contraction and relaxation in wavelike movements; in other words, peristalsis.

Smooth muscles need energy to contract as well. Intestinal muscles produce their own contraction-energy. The vital detail here is the following: although we consider contraction to require energy, we never take into consideration that relaxation requires it as well. *In fact, relaxation requires more energy than contraction. When we simply take a look at the biochemistry of contraction of muscles, calcium entering the cell induces contraction. For relaxation, calcium needs to be extracted from the cell. This requires a lot of energy.*

Extracting calcium is much more difficult than absorbing it. For example, calcium canal brokers that are blood pressure drugs prevent hypertension by blocking calcium from accessing the cell. Hypertension means hyper-contraction. What I'm trying to say is that hypertension is something similar to the "constipation of the vein."

Calcium's antidote is magnesium.

- **hypertension**: vein contraction

- **cramps**: muscles remaining contracted
- **fibromyalgia**: contraction of back muscles; being unable to relax
- **headache**: tense, contracted neck muscles
- **teeth grinding**: contraction of jaw muscles

Smooth muscles contract when constipated. Therefore, it is possible to grasp how a simple magnesium supplement could make things easier for these problems.

So why can't intestinal muscles find the required energy to extract calcium? Here are the reasons:

- If mitochondria are damaged, they generate low amounts of ATP via glycolysis.
- It's out of the question to burn fat and generate high levels of energy unless SCFA is produced, fiber is consumed, and there are some beneficial bacteria.
- In case of no fermentation, they cannot find enough energy, since they cannot provide extra electrons from the new and beneficial bacteria in order to generate sufficient ATP.
- If no plant-based nutrients are consumed, then they cannot find magnesium for laxation. Magnesium is in the center of the plant. The center of chlorophyll is

magnesium. If there are no fibrous, colorful, vivid plants consumed, then our source of magnesium is limited.

Intestinal movements are circadian, just like the entire digestive system. They slow down at night and accelerate during the day. We all have experienced how it is difficult to digest food that is consumed at night. Hence, in reference to intestinal health, in addition to eating, not eating is also an option. *In most recent studies, it has been found that the repair capacity of stem cells in the intestines is doubled during a one-day-long nutrient starvation.*

One-layered cells in the intestines are regenerated every five days—they have a short lifespan. How are they regenerated? At the bottom of the villus, the intestinal stem cells wait; when the ends get damaged, they take their place to repair. But, with age and the increasing affects of malnutrition, stem cell capacity gradually decreases. After a certain point, intestines cannot function properly with all the damaged cells. This is one of the causes of leaky gut I've been discussing.

Clinical studies show that after twenty-four hours of nutrient starvation, the metabolism of intestinal stem cells change. *Stem cells mainly utilize glucose. However, during a long period of nutrient starvation, they make a metabolic shift into burning fat. This enhances their capacity to do work and doubles their capacity to repair.*

This study is new and only focuses on intestinal stem cells; but even so, we can apply this idea to all the stem cells of all the tissues and hope that nutrient starvation will renew them. And at this point, in order to sustain a periodic nutrient starvation, it makes sense to begin fasting at 5:00 in the evening until 9:00 in the morning for sixteen hours, in line with the circadian rhythm. Stem cells are Day Zero cells. They are spotless and brand new. We can reset and regenerate as far as our Day Zero cells. It seems that the path goes through fasting at night.

I've been continuously emphasizing the significance of fasting at night. So now, let's respond to "what do we eat during the day?"

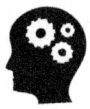

Chapter 5:

"Gather the sun for me." —Zülfü Livaneli

The Basics of Healthy Eating: Plant-Based Nutrients

In three of the books I published, I gave detailed information on what constitutes as healthy food. Here, instead of making a list of foods, I will examine the topic with a different perspective. Nevertheless, ultimately, all roads lead to Rome—in other words, to vital plant-based nutrients and fats.

The vitality of nutrients is a wide enough topic to write book about. When sunlight reached the earth, plants found a way to gather that light and convert it into electrons—the process we know as photosynthesis. Since that day, they implicitly pass it on to us and to animals by way of nutrients.

In my previous book, *Quantum Mitochondrial Diet (Kuantum Beslenme)*, my purpose was to explain the importance of photosynthesis for vitality. While the photosynthesis-nutrition connection proves that living beings feed on light, we now know that we should also take circadian rhythms into consideration every time the word "light" is mentioned. **Plants are also circadian. They gather electrons during the day; at night, they store them as glucose in their fruits and roots.**

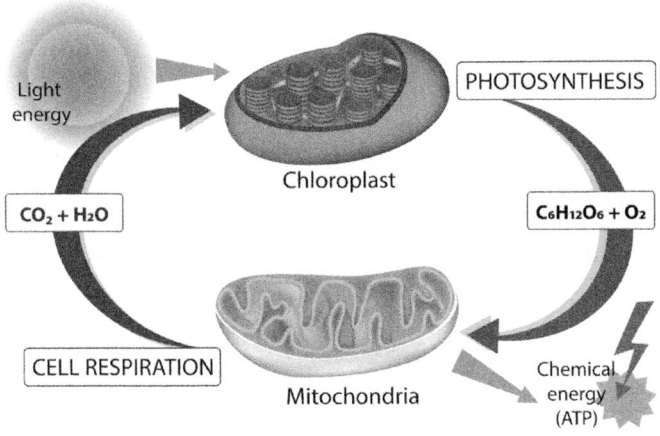

The electrons that belong to the hydrogen in H2O of the water drawn from the earth disintegrate with sunlight. These one-of-a-kind beings that generate energy by prying the electrons from water with the help of light transport these electrons to their own ETC. This is exactly the way we carry the electrons from food to our ETC. Instead of our NADH, plants have NADPH to transport their electrons. The electrons formed by the sunlight and water in plants are collected in NADPH. When we consume plants, we take in the plant's electrons and NADPH. This is the main benefit of plants.

We also, generally, have NADPH in our bodies. NADPH works as an electron carrier in our bodies. Its electrons are not converted into energy; they are used as antioxidants. In every procedure where there is oxidation—in other words, where prevention of rusting is necessary—NADPH is used as an electron donor. Its molecule deserves all the given terms such as antioxidant, electron-giver, and alkali-maker.

In that case, NADPH is friends with "whoever" deals with the free radicals undertaking oxidation. NADPH is the main helper for all internal cellular systems that dispose of free radicals. The electron inside is not used in order to be converted into energy, such as with NADH and FADH; it is used as antioxidant. As a matter of fact, the main purpose of our antioxidant systems is to provide more electrons. Glutathione, the master antioxidant, detoxifies through the donation of its electrons. Once it donates its electrons as antioxidants, NADPH replaces the electrons that were lost in order to be reduced—in other words, to be charged. *NADPH is the one that charges glutathione— our main detoxifying substance—when it finishes.*

The main component from which NADPH is

generated is called D-ribose. D-ribose provides assistance by producing NADPH in the detoxification system of the liver. NADPH produced from ribose cleanses the glutathione. As the toxin load increases in the body, and as the poor quality food penetrating the mitochondria increases the amount of free radicals, the need for NADPH also increases. That's why in almost all diseases, it's very important to change to a plant-based diet. Perhaps sentences such as "as we eat plants, we receive more antioxidants" now have a stronger seat in your mind. Plants are reducers. Plants are antioxidants. Plants are filled with electron charges such as NADPH. They charge us as we eat them!

Our glutathione reserves are not infinite. They decrease gradually as a result of toxins, malnutrition, chemicals, stress, insomnia, and alcohol intake. Aging itself is a condition of glutathione deficiency. Even for a small spot on the skin, we can point to glutathione—the main cleaner—being diminished due to aging. It is called an age spot, after all. Any disease in any part of the body—from the brain to the joints, from skin to the endocrine glands—are the result of wastes accumulating in the body as one ages. If we add to eating habits that generate waste not adapting to the circadian rhythm as well as insufficient cleaning, we would get a clearer picture.

The purpose of recommending the abundant consumption of plants—namely vegetables, fruits, spices, legumes, and nuts—is mainly for obtaining clean electrons. Plants generate less free radicals while burning at the ETC, and they clean their own wastes with the electrons they bring with them. In short, the answer to the question of "what shall we eat?" can simply be summarized as "mostly plant-based foods."

Of course, in order to preserve their vitality, it is important to eat plant-based foods that are raw and seasonal.

Plants are also circadian; since they have a biorhythm, summer plants hold the wavelengths of summer sunlight within them. Likewise, winter plants belong to the winter, and they express that. There is data traffic between plants and humans.

All plant-based foods, vegetables, fruits, spices, legumes, nuts, greens, and so on… each and every one of them carry light.

Let's make a small note here: darker colored plants contain more sunlight. As it is with us when we sunbathe and our skin turns a darker color, plants that have darkened in color contain more of the above-mentioned NADPH electrons. "Suntanned" plants are preferred. There is a wide color scale from black to brown, purple, blue, red, orange, yellow, and white.

In most plants, vegetables and fruits, the outer shells are darker than the inside and richer in antioxidants. Take eggplant as an example. If we consider its outer shell as the skin, its dark color indicates that it contains more light. Another significant aspect of plants following their color and vitality is the valuable fats they contain. The more fatty the plant, the better it is. For example, olives are dark in color; they are fatty; and, they are a plants. Nigella seeds, sesame seeds, and flaxseeds are brown, black, fatty; and, they are plants. I believe you get the gist of it.

Sea plants, seaweed, and algae should also be considered to be in the category of plants. From algae, let's move on to other creatures in the sea. Let's take a look at the fish.

For a healthy diet, fatty fish are especially highly recommended. The reason is due to the omega-3 fatty acids they contain. The omega fatty acid found in seafood is DHA, which is crucial for cell membranes. DHA of all cell membranes, including mitochondria membrane as well, should be protected. Moreover, high doses of DHA supplements should also be taken. I would like to emphasize the importance of DHA and the forgotten vitamin E supplements for protecting the eyes from blue light. Protecting the eyes is protecting the circadian clock.

Membranes are the first place to get hit by the free radical damage in the cell. Free radicals first damage the inner cell membrane of the mitochondria. It's where they are generated; when the membrane is pierced, leaky mitochondria condition takes place and damages the outer membrane of the cell.

Do not be shocked by all this detailed information. You will come across phrases such as "seventy percent of our brain consists of fat"; you will feel the need to acquire information about fats and membranes. What these phrases try to convey is that another way of protecting cell membranes from free radical damage is to send in new raw materials to repair the damaged parts—namely good fats and antioxidants.

Free radicals decrease the amount of electrons on the membranes. In medicine, we call this lipid peroxidation. To put it simply, let's say it's the cell membrane rusting. In my book *We are Full but Starving (Tokuz ama Açız)*, I discuss the importance of the cell membranes in detail. Let's write down the term *cell membrane* as *cell mem-brain*. In other words, the membrane of the cell is its brain!

In previous chapters, I explained why it is important for the mitochondria inner membrane to remain intact. I hope that by now you know the following: the ETC is on the inner membrane of the mitochondria; electrons flow over the membrane; if the electron flow is clogged, free radical damage oxidizes the membrane; oxidation tears the membrane; cytochrome C leaking outside drives the cell to the point of no return, which is the beginning of all degenerative diseases and cancer. No disease begins unless there is leaky mitochondria. Your general health and your mitochondria health are one and the same.

In order to take an analytical approach to health, you need to comprehend well the algorithms of cause and effect. In "The Ultimate 5" section, I tried to explain the biochemistry of it all in detail and as simply as I possibly can. Now, let's have a look at our night life. According to the circadian rhythm, what does "night" actually mean? Let's find out its meaning for our bodies and for our health.

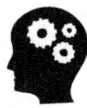

Why Do We Sleep?

"No small art is it to sleep: It is necessary for that purpose to keep awake all day." —Friedrich Nietzsche

As you read these words, I don't know whether it is day or night; but there is one thing that I do know for certain. Many sleep researchers are losing sleeping over trying to figure out why we sleep. Therefore, it is obviously of great importance.

Let me ask you the following: How many nights did you sleep well in the last week? When was the last time you woke up according to your internal clock, cheerful and energetic, without having to set your alarm clock to wake you up? If you are dismayed with the first question, and your reply to the second question is "I don't remember," you're not alone.

Almost two thirds of adults cannot sleep the recommended eight hours per night. This may not be a surprise to you. But, I am certain it will unpleasantly shock you to learn about all the heavy costs of insomnia, and its disruption of the circadian rhythm. For instance, I can tell you that those who regularly sleep less than seven hours have twice the risk of cancer; or, I can tell you that sleep deprivation is listed in Alzheimer's etiology. Furthermore, only one week of sleep deprivation or irregular sleep is enough to interrupt your blood sugar levels; and, it could lead you to pre-diabetic blood test results. I can also remind you that insufficient sleep is among the perpetrators of heart diseases; it is also a trigger for psychological conditions, such as depression and anxiety. The list goes on and on.

Although you won't immediately get ill as a consequence of insomnia, you probably will notice how you crave more food on the days you feel exhausted following a sleepless night. When you do not get a good night's sleep and cannot rest, the craving for carbohydrates increases. In a nutshell, a shorter amount of sleep means a shorter life. The party-lovers' "we'll get to sleep when we die" statement turns into a self-fulfilling prophecy.

The World Health Organization (WHO) states that sleep deprivation is an epidemic in modern, industrialized countries. The US, UK, Japan, and South Korea take the lead. However, others shouldn't want to compete with these countries where sleep deprivation and its related diseases are skyrocketing. I certainly believe we are living in times when my fellow colleagues should be prescribing sleep. It is a pain-free, ache-free, easy, and pleasant prescription. Moreover, there are no side effects. Yet, the greatest problem of this era is the prescribing of sleeping pills, which has become convention instead of prescribing sleep. The reason we are socially apathetic towards sleep issues and pushing our limits with sleep deficiency is perhaps because we do not yet comprehend the severity of it in medical terms.

Sleep is still a biological enigma guarding most of its secrets; but for now, let's focus on the benefits of sleep as far as we know.

Benefits of Sleep

Why do we sleep? The simplest answer is one that is also the most accurate for this era—to charge our batteries. It's just like our mobile phones; or, with the rest of our electrical appliances. By taking a deeper perspective, we could also claim the following: we sleep to take *full* advantage of the darkness of night. In the dark, in the night lies great benefits. Sleep is definitely not a waste of time; on the contrary, it's an asset.

First and foremost, we sleep to reset our brains. Sleep calibrates the emotional pathways in our brains. We sleep so that on the following day we can steer our social lives and emotions in the right direction. The brain's lymphatic system detoxifies the metabolism wastes inside the brain throughout the night. We sleep in order to have a cleaner brain. Sleep strengthens the immune system. It enhances the fight against tumors and aids in the resistance against infections. Sleep balances the metabolism of sugar, insulin, and leptin. On the other hand, sleep deprivation causes weight gain.

At night, our intestinal microbiota goes through a different kind of balancing. A good night's sleep at the right times is a *must* for healthy intestinal microbiota as well. All beneficial bacteria in our bodies adapt to this circadian rhythm. Bacteria active during the day and bacteria active at night are different.

The unwanted bacteria and viruses are also destroyed at night, when the immune system is active. We know that sleep deprivation or sleeping late at night weakens the immune system, and that we catch the flu very easily after jet lag. If we catch a cold or the flu, we are commonly so exhausted that we can't even lift a finger. At times like these, the immune system wants to put itself in sleep mode in order to empower itself. We want to lay down and sleep. That's what the body requests of us.

Sleep is the greatest immunity defense. Natural melatonin is the strongest antioxidant. Even just one night of insufficient and poor sleep harms a person— just like a poor quality meal does. Perhaps, it's even more harmful than a poor quality meal. However, don't be stressed if you are sleep deprived, as sleep deprivation is already a cause for biological stress.

Cause of Stress: Sleep Deprivation

Chronobiology—a scientific field focusing on time and health—explores biorhythms, which are tuned in to daylight. According to chronobiology, we should go to bed at 11:00 p.m. and avoid the light of all electronic devices at least three hours before doing so. I'm sure you've already heard how electromagnetic pollution has influenced the rise of modern day diseases, especially the chronic ones. That's why your mobile phone is not welcome in your bedroom. Come to think of it, it's quite easy to grasp the fact that the light coming from our mobile phones—which we check in the middle of the night—shock our internal clocks; in other words, our biorhythms, which operate with light.

Two things that we do at night disrupt the circadian rhythm: eating and having contact with electronic devices. When we undertake these activities, our repair time and hormone rhythms are interrupted, and we are defeated in our race against time.

Our biological clocks start with the secretion of cortisol with the dawn of day. The moment cortisol is released, melatonin stops. For the rest of the day, as cortisol levels decrease, hormones that boost our energy levels and feelings of happiness, such as serotonin and adrenaline, are produced. As the day turns to night, serotonin turns into melatonin. As of 11:00 p.m., melatonin peaks and the time for sleep arrives; where there is sleep, there can be no cortisol. When it gets darker, we sleep with melatonin; to the morning light, we wake up with cortisol, and then continue with serotonin and adrenalin throughout the day. This is what the hormone cycle is like.

We know that cortisol is the stress hormone. In short-term states of stress, it is desired and normal that cortisol rises. It is customary for cortisol to wake us up in the mornings, like an alarm clock. In an emergency situation, even if we are hungry, cortisol increases the blood sugar levels at once and generates the energy required to handle that emergency. These are all normal.

However, we should never wish for cortisol to be secreted continuously—that is, chronically. That kind of stress is harmful. When it is recommended for you to manage your stress, it is cortisol that is being referred to, as it creates chronic low-levels of stress. While mentioning diseases caused by low levels of chronic stress, we should also remember that their effects can be reduced by living in tune with the circadian rhythm.

The system operating in the body at times of stress is called the sympathetic system, whereas the system that steps in at times of relaxation is called parasympathetic. *Cortisol is the hormone of the sympathetic system, while melatonin is the hormone of the parasympathetic system. Both of these systems operate in cycles; they are circadian. The sympathetic system is active all day long, and the parasympathetic is active at night.*

The parasympathetic system is the system that

manages the internal organs. Repair and renewal is under the control of this system. More active during the night, this system prepares the grounds for repair processes that take place while we're sleeping. If we do not bring our circadian rhythms into a state where the parasympathetic system can become active at night, we will then have chronic stress in our bodies. Since our biorhythms adjust to light, if we go to bed late every night, the repair mechanism will shut down.

It is an obvious survival mechanism that the body adjusts itself to the sun, which is the most reliable source of external time. Although this is the main mechanism in adjusting our internal clocks, our daily routines are also taken into consideration. Besides daylight, our daily routines such as meal times, hours of activity, and sleep times affect our internal clocks as well. How do our daily lives and habits affect the circadian rhythm? Let's see.

Lifestyles and the Internal Clock

Jet Lag

The most common disrupter of our internal clocks is jet lag, which occurs as a result of time zone differences. Recovering from jet lag, which we experience after long flights, actually takes longer than we think. Our internal clocks are not that easy to reset; because the internal clock indicator in our brains—the SCN center—can make readjustments only for one hour per day. This means that after jet lag, to get used to the time zone of wherever we are, we need as many days as the difference in time. If there is a five-hour difference, then it will take five days for our internal clocks to readjust to the external time. The main reason for jet lag is long flights; but even drinking coffee might have a jet lag effect. Let's call this coffee jet lag.

Coffee Jet Lag

When we consume coffee in the evenings, our sleep is less effective, we sleep later than usual, and our melatonin levels decrease. Thus, coffee is also a disrupter of the circadian internal clock. There are special coffee detox-genes in the liver, which disposes of coffee. They vary from person to person; they may work faster or more slowly. For some people, even after drinking coffee in the evenings, it is still easy to fall asleep; for others, coffee consumed early in the morning may prevent sleep later in the evening. Between these two, there is a genetic difference in the detox enzymes. Despite this difference, the disposal of coffee from the body also slows down with age. We should be aware of caffeine jet lag. At least try to prefer decaffeinated coffee after 2:00 p.m.

Now that coffee is our topic, let's talk about how it drives sleep away.

It Goes Back to ATP

Feeling sleepy happens in two ways. First, as it gets darker, the darkness signal produces melatonin in the pineal gland. Melatonin is also called the vampire hormone, because of its relation to darkness. Second, we feel sleepy because the body's batteries become run-down. In other words, our mitochondrial energy becomes run-down.

On nights after a long and exhausting day, even

with the lights on, we cannot resist sleep; we find it difficult to keep our eyes open, and we literally doze off.

It is due to the substance called adenosine, which accumulates in the brain.

The accumulation of adenosine puts us to sleep. So, what is adenosine? It's the "A" in ATP, adenosine triphosphate.

When we use three phosphates of ATP, we are down to ADP (adenosine two phosphates); after using that as well, we are down to AMP (adenosine monophosphate). When we use the final phosphate, we are left with adenosine. No phosphate means empty batteries.

Fatigue is conveyed to the brain when adenosine levels increase in the blood. In order to be able to convey this, there are receptors that connect with adenosine to be able to determine how much adenosine is accumulated in the brain. When adenosine receptors in the brain are filled with adenosine, it is inevitable that we fall asleep. What happens is coffee connects to adenosine receptors in the brain, before adenosine does. It delays the sleep signals and provides a fake wakefulness and energy. It is true that coffee awakens and energizes those who occasionally drink coffee. Those who often consume coffee have desensitized receptors. In time, their need for coffee gradually intensifies.

The presence of adenosine tells us that the AMP/ADP/ATP balance has broken down, and that there is no raw material to produce new ATP. In order to take a break from this exhaustion, the body puts you to sleep. In this state, you cannot generate ATP even if you eat, because it takes a long time for the battery at the AMP level to be charged. D-ribose is the nutritional supplement that helps AMP to turn into ADP. In case of an emergency, D-ribose might be considered in place of coffee to give us energy. In addition to coffee, tea, energy drinks, chocolate, and some painkillers also delay sleep.

Social Jet Lag

Then there is social jet lag. We usually stay up late when we socialize with friends. Of course, how often you do this is your prerogative. But please do not neglect to get the rest that your body deserves. You must—for a healthy and long life. Now, let's move onto another crucial cause of jet lag.

Electronic Digital Jet Leg

In my opinion, this is the most significant type of jet lag among the ones discussed. The reason is everyone— young and elderly—is consumed by television and other electronic devices, day and night. Even the lamplight in our houses is an internal clock disrupter. However, electronics are at the top of the list.

The electronic devices you use at night are a real source for chronic cellular stress, as they **instigate cortisol secretion.** Light coming from their screens prevent melatonin secretion. If there's no melatonin at the required time, then cortisol becomes active. Cortisol immediately changes the eating behavior and tends to increase blood sugar levels. It makes you eat more; it makes you feel hungry. You must have heard friends say the following: "I'm taking cortisone, and I gained a lot of weight." In short, I cannot think of anything more ideal than candlelight and light coming from a fireplace. On the other hand, electronic devices have blue light.

Blue Light

Our eyes are not merely for seeing. There are receptors in the eye that evaluate the time of day. The retina of the eye is like a camera. It measures precisely the daylight spectrum. The light seen contains the entire color spectrum of the rainbow. The main colors are blue, green, and red. When they are combined, they form white light, which is the sunlight. It is a light of wavelengths between 400-700 nanometers that can be seen. Every color has its own wavelength within this spectrum. Red has the longest, and purple has the shortest wavelength.

Besides the receptors of the eyes that enable them to see, the receptors that adjust the circadian rhythm are crucial for health. They are photoreceptors called melanopsin. Their task is not to perceive shapes but to determine the wavelengths from the color of sunlight about the time of day, so that they can inform the center in the brain that actually measures time. The actual center measuring time—the SCN, also known as suprachiasmatic nucleus—is in the hypothalamus; it is our biological clock. It's a zeitgeber, a biorhythm pacemaker.

The SCN is known as the master clock. The SCN collaborates with the brain and all of the organs. It maintains the circadian rhythm of the organs and indicates the times of hormone secretion. The SCN is the clock adjusting the secretion of the growth hormone from the pituitary gland, melatonin from the pineal gland, cortisol from the adrenal glands, the thyroid hormone from the thyroid gland, and sex hormones from the gonads. Those who have Alzheimer's confuse the time of day, the year, whether they are hungry or not, due to the degeneration of the SCN.

Melanopsin carrying light data to the SCN is especially sensitive to blue light. The wavelength blue light is between 400-500 nm (480). We could say melanopsin is a photopigment. It's the pigment that also regulates the biorhythm for the visually impaired; it's the pigment that catches the light. It serves the circadian rhythm, not vision. Melanopsin informs the SCN of the sleep-wake time, and it immediately shares this with the entire body.

There are studies that show that the dopamine hormone assists melanopsin during circadian adjustments. At this point, we can connect wintertime depression called SAD to decreasing dopamine levels.

Since melanopsin is sensitive to the wavelengths of blue light, it proves we're right when we say that the blue light of electronics is unhealthy. Mobile devices, laptops, computers, and the TV all emit blue light between 400-500 nm.

Perceiving the wavelengths even after it's dark, melanopsin is unable to recognize it's in the night phase of the circadian rhythm. Thinking it's still daytime, melanopsin informs this to the SCN, and through the SCN to the entire body. Yet, I've been explaining throughout this book that different functions take place during the day and at night.

It's not considered to be a serious health issue so far. Even if it seems as though a couple of nights like this is not of any real concern, according to a study, people spend eighty-seven percent of their days inside their homes or offices. Therefore, we are always harassed by the blue light. It's fine at the office; but in the evenings when you come home, if you are still looking at your electronics, the circadian rhythm confuses the signals.

The blue light coming from our electronic devices is almost an inseparable part of our current lives. Many studies have been undertaken concerning the damage that the blue light has on our health. It seems this topic will be an important one for medicine in the future.

Melanopsin electronic blue light is also transmitted from the eye to the SCN. With the information received from the SCN, the pineal gland is told not to produce melatonin, or the sleep hormone. Although other colors are also influential, it is the blue light that is mostly emitted by electronics and that stimulates the SCN. Red light does not change this situation that much either. It is smart that night lamps are designed to emit an orange-red light, so that sleep is not disturbed.

Blue light is a stress-builder only when it gets to the eyes at night, not during the day. Blue light increases the levels of the stress hormone cortisol and decreases melatonin. Cortisol decreases the functioning of the parasympathetic system, which is the reset system. However, nighttime and sleep is the time for the parasympathetic system and regeneration.

Blue light especially affects the energy metabolism, because it's circadian. Insulin, glucagon, leptin, ghrelin, all of these hormones related to food and satiation are circadian. The liver, the pancreas, the intestines, and the entire digestive system are circadian as well. Blue light keeps these hormones with the rhythm, day and night.

As I've said, when you eat is more important than what you eat. Blue light stimulates your appetite at night. We know that night eaters are more prone to weight problems, and more inclined towards diseases such as hypertriglyceridemia, hypercholesterolemia, elevated uric acid, diabetes, and insulin resistance. The pancreas also has melatonin receptors. Glucagon receptors, which have the opposite effect of insulin, are sensitive to melatonin. If melatonin is not present, insulin is activated.

Hence, the perpetrator of your nighttime-snacking is electronics, which prevent melatonin from shutting down the system. An hour of exposure to blue light reduces melatonin by sixty percent. Insufficient melatonin—in other words, the decline in sleep efficiency—is associated with weight issues, psychiatric conditions, and cancer. *In short, blue light and eating at night disrupts the circadian rhythm.*

It is wise to sleep with a mask; to use blackout curtains; to keep the television, computers, and mobile devices out of the bedroom; to avoid contact with electronic devices three to four hours prior to sleep; and to protect your eyes against this light.

If we remember that the SCN is a *timekeeper*, then we know that the circadian cycle is shortened and not the twenty-four hour period that it ought to be:

- when there's light at night,
- when we are awake at night, and
- when we eat at night.

We can understand better through the logic of accelerated cycles that we will be fast forwarding our own biological time and age more quickly if we eat at night and stay awake under the light. Perhaps, since the entire world is shining with bright lights, we all feel like time is moving faster.

Consequentially, in order to support the biological timekeeper, live long, be fit, remain healthy and young, we need to sleep on time, avoid eating at night, and avoid being exposed to light—which destroys melatonin.

Melatonin speaks for itself; it is the *sleep* hormone. It is secreted in the dark. So, under daylight and pseudo-light, the secretion stops. When there is no melatonin, there is cortisol. This means the following:

- If there's cortisol, the body is under stress.
- Blue light is a cause for chronic stress.
- Blue light is a cause for cortisol.
- Blue light interferes with the circadian internal clock.
- Blue light is a great danger for all of us, especially children.
- Not only electronics, but LED lights and wi-fi are also harmful.
- The best choice is candlelight or the fireplace.

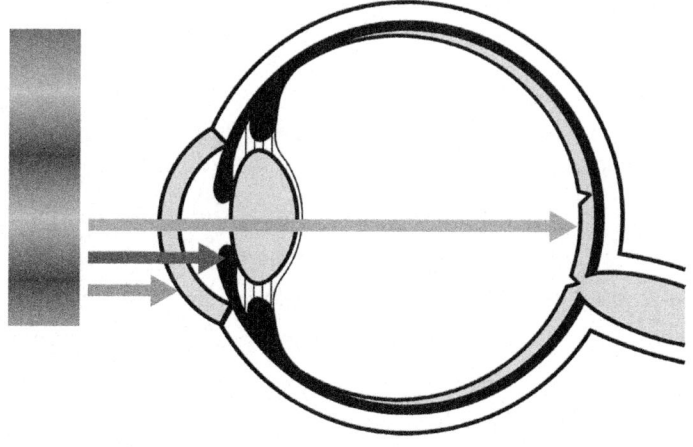

Malillumination: New Disease of the Era

Edison invented the light bulb, and melatonin stopped functioning. Of course, Edison is not to be blamed for the invention of the century; but let's face it, if the melatonin hormone could speak, it would probably say that Edison is the one it hates the most. The reason being that our circadian rhythm was disrupted with the invention of the light bulb. And with the electric devices we are exposed to nowadays, it has made its peak.

Let's call being exposed to unwelcome light or not being exposed to sufficient daylight *malillumination*. *Mal* means bad, and *illumination* is light. I believe we should add this to the "widespread diseases we are unaware of" list of our era. I assume I do not need to remind you that those who work on the night shift, who travel often and have jet lag, and who wake up for their children in the middle of the night, have disrupted circadian rhythms.

I'm not referring to those nights where it's inevitable that we miss out on sleep. What I am referring to is the rhythm disruptions we purposely cause for ourselves. If we go to bed late voluntarily, if we eat at odd hours, we can change these habits. If we do not, we will age sooner than expected, as our circadian rhythms will be accelerated. In fact, the entire world lives today as if someone pressed the fast forward button. As a result, people age before their time and more quickly. We have to put a stop to this!

Our Quantum Biology

Since the topic is light and its effects on our health, let's recall that light is a quantum phenomena, and that quantum biology has a role in all this. Light is a subject of quantum biology. We cannot define circadian rhythm with Newtonian physics and classical biology. When we enter the world of quantum physics and quantum biology, then we can grasp the idea that we are in contact with the entire universe, not just the sun. This perspective is way beyond what we already know about health. However, once we start talking about the sun and the circadian rhythm of day and night, then we can start really discussing this topic. Everything is bound by the rules of nature and quantum biology of the universe.

The sunlight comes in packs of photons. In this pack, the energy of light is called *quant*. It can show features of waves and particles at the same time. The photon is an energy-pack as much as it's a light-pack. Light, heat, mass gravity—these three control the entire biology.

We know that the rising of the sun is the primary clock that gives a start to our biological rhythms. *The sun synchronizes us with the universe, with itself, and all other living beings.* Humans, plants, animals, fungi, bacteria, and even planktons included—all living creatures follow this adjustment. It is a matter of survival. Finding food, reproduction, famine and abundance, efforts to survive—they all take place in accordance with the light. Light always creates a chemical event wherever it shows itself. It ignites the spark for chemical occurrences. Photosynthesis is proof of this. Our production of vitamin D is another proof of this. However, this system should be circadian. Where there is no sun, there should be no light.

All living creatures are connected with each other. This is called quantum entanglement. All life is bound to one another through flows of energy. All is one. We are all bound to each other, to the Moon, to the Sun, and to the whole universe. The Sun, the Moon and universe consist of photon-light, magnetism, and mass gravity. In other words, our biology consists of photon-light, magnetism, and mass gravity as well. In order to perceive light among these three factors connecting us to the whole, we have sensors in our body—in our eyes, on our skin, in our bloodstream, and even *in the fibrils of our DNA*. I think everything inside the microcosm cell and the macrocosm universe are connected to one another through light.

To synchronize ourselves and our bodies with the universe, we have to set our wristwatches to the time of the sun. Perhaps, we will have places to travel to, not drug names, written on future prescriptions. In some parts of the world, the wavelengths of the sun are more ideal; so they may give you prescriptions accordingly. Your doctor may say, "well, it's probably best if you go and live in this X city to preserve your circadian rhythm…"

For now, keep the above in your mind as futuristic medical tips. In the meantime, let's just make an effort to protect our eating-fasting, sleep-wake, and light-darkness cycles. Rhythms, cycles, flows—they all should be in harmony. They should have an order. That's the central theme of this book.

I hope you have gained a brand new perspective through this book about how to protect your health and lead a happy and long life. This book is not here to make you count the calories; it's a book to provide you with good habits. Before I finish, I would like to thank you for showing the patience to read and understand this book

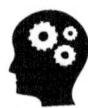

Some Tips So That You Won't Be Bound to Pills All Your Life

HOW TO SET YOUR CIRCADIAN RHYTHM:

- Wake up early in the mornings. Before 7:30 a.m., try to look directly at the daylight out of your window. This sets the circadian clock. It's the quickest way to obtain the dopamine (pleasure) hormone. The amount of your melatonin secretion that evening will increase, and you will sleep much better. If you suffer from insomnia, first, you should wake up early and go out to set your clock. This will prevent you from walking around with a foggy mind, and feeling sleepy all day long. Also, you will struggle less with sleep deprivation at night.
- If you cannot do this, looking at a

melatonin lamp will also help (a melatonin lamp consists of all wavelengths of the daylight).

- Do not wear sunglasses when sunlight does not bother you.
- Avoid TV, your mobile phone and laptop, and computer light at night.
- You should avoid contact with the above devices at least two hours prior to sleep. Do not keep them in your bedroom, either.
- Use a screen filter on your computer and mobile phone.
- They already have built-in blue light filters. Turn them on at night.
- Do not use LED lights at home. Prefer a red light, fireplace, or candlelight. You may also find daylight lamps.
- Turn down the lights in your room at least one hour before you go to sleep.
- Try to completely protect your eyes from light when sleeping with a sleep mask and/or curtains.
- Do not set the temperature very high in your bedroom. Keep it low while you are sleeping. Falling asleep in a cool room helps the circadian rhythm.
- Do not look at your electronic devices if you wake up in the middle of the night.

How to Increase the Number of Mitochondria:

- Exercise regularly.
- Have more contact with the cold.
- In order to increase the number of brown fat tissue, which multiplies in the cold, take a cold shower before you go out.
- Use mitochondria supplements.
- Try to keep up with nighttime nutrient starvation; apply the system at least a few days a week.
- Try avoiding the consumption of simple carbohydrates, especially in the evenings.
- Limit your alcohol intake.
- Be certain to ask your doctor before using any medications.
- Beware of environmental toxins such as pesticides, cigarettes, etc.
- Try to breathe well. If you suffer from a deviated septum, snoring, or sleep apnea, look for a solution so that you can breathe right. Find ways to remain calm if you suffer from anxiety; remember that anxiety creates a lack of oxygen.

Recommendations About Nutrition:

- In the morning, eat mostly proteins; at lunchtime, eat complex carbohydrates; and for supper, eat fats and vegetables.
- Try to stop eating around 5:00-6:00 p.m.

- Try to consume natural, seasonal, and organic food.
- Tend to eat more raw food as opposed to cooked food.
- Chew at least twenty times for every bite.
- Watch your consumption of fats.
- Keep in mind that instead of consuming poor quality food, it's better in the long-term to remain hungry.

Life Suggestions:

- Meditate.
- Live with mindfulness and conscious awareness.
- Try to be in nature as much as you can.
- Make an effort to be in contact with the earth.
- Have a pet.
- Sleep well.
- Try to keep social jet lag limited to two days per week.
- Do not consume coffee after 2:00 p.m.

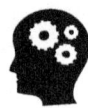

Epilogue

MY PERSONAL RECOMMENDATION FOR SURVIVAL: TRAIN YOURSELF

Are you aware of the tremendous effort that is made worldwide in protecting our health, living a long life, or even trying to attain immortality? Do you know where the world is headed? Perhaps, you will feel as if you're reading a science-fiction scenario when you read what I'm about to tell you. But it's all true!

You can become younger by switching your blood with younger blood. And, this is legal! In China, babies with planned genes have been born. These babies were allegedly planned to eliminate diseased genes; but then, it appeared that the same gene was affecting the brain capacity as well. In other words, the first super-modified humans were generated!

- With a 3D printer, spare organs are being made.

- Through 5G-technology, surgeries are being performed by robots, internationally.
- Procedures that make you swallow a pipe, such as an endoscopy, are now possible through having you swallow tiny nano robots.
- Watson computers makes diagnoses now more quickly than doctors.
- Wearable technologies now inform your doctor about your blood sugar, directly through the watch on your wrist.
- There are groundbreaking stem cell remedies taking place.
- There are exclusive devices and drugs for cancer treatment.
- Personalized immunotherapies are being created.
- Plans are being made to freeze the entire body before it is dead by cryopreservation, to be revived years later.
- It's only a matter of time before we go to Mars for sightseeing!

And while all of these are happening, the world population is increasing constantly. Will food resources be sufficient for everyone? As nutritional values of food are spoiled, diseases will increase. Do you think the whole population will be able to benefit from the technologies mentioned above equally? I'm sorry to say this, but thinking that would be naive more than anything else. As all those who can benefit from these types of futuristic and inevitably expensive methods and head toward immortality, what do you think will happen to those who are unable to benefit? Will they lead short and morbid lives? Or, will people be segregated according to their states of health as well?

Let me tell you where I think the world is swiftly heading toward: the "health Elites" are coming. Health elites! People who have the means to benefit from the technologies I mentioned above, as well as the ones I do not yet know about, for their own longevity and health. Have you seen the movies Gattaca and Elysium?

Watch them if you haven't. You will see clues in them about the future.

So, what are we to do then? We will also be one of the health elites! All of my books were written to turn you into data elites; to enable you to compete with the opportunities of health elites on your own. We too are in the race, armed with our knowledge! What they buy you will obtain with what you know, by not getting ill at all. In order to lead a healthy and long life, knowledge is more valuable than money! Learning how to be healthy is our greatest ammunition. We will opt for not getting sick at all. Can anyone see any other options?

Printed in Great Britain
by Amazon

41397762R00106